Telepathy in the Clinical Process

Telepathy in the Clinical Process explores telepathy as it appears in the psychoanalytic process, both in contemporary practice and in historical contexts.

The contributors explore striking dynamic and clinical data in considering how telepathy can express itself in transference and countertransference, its profound effect on psychoanalysts, and its frequent role in helping patients in treatment. From a wide range of theoretical persuasions – relational, Bionian, Winnicottian, contemporary Freudian – each author explores this phenomenon. Focused on the clinical process, the book contains examples from the contributors' own practice throughout.

Telepathy in the Clinical Process will be of great interest to psychoanalysts in practice and in training. It will also be relevant to academics and students of psychoanalytic studies and parapsychology.

Richard Reichbart, Ph.D., is a Fellow and Training Analyst at the Institute for Psychoanalytic Training and Research, a component society of the International Psychoanalytic Association. He has published extensively on psychoanalysis and maintains a private psychology practice in Ho-Ho-Kus, New Jersey.

"This collection stands as a remarkable contribution to the ongoing dialogue between psychoanalysis and parapsychology. The authors' commitment to exploring telepathy and its implications for clinical practice is both courageous and thought-provoking, challenging traditional boundaries and encouraging fresh perspectives. By weaving together historical context, theoretical innovation, and vivid clinical examples, the book invites readers to reconsider the depth and complexity of the analyst–patient relationship. I recommend this work for anyone seeking to expand their understanding of the mind's hidden potential and the transformative possibilities within psychoanalytic treatment."

Stanley Krippner, Ph.D., Research Professor, California Institute for Human Sciences

"Based on a remarkable two-day international teleconference on Telepathy sponsored by IPTAR in NYC, this book is a worthy sequel to George Devereux's (1953) classic, *Psychoanalysis and the Occult*. This rich collection combines research of leading clinicians, theorists and historians on the intriguing and ever controversial subject of 'thought transference.' Recurring but always unexpected, telepathy is sometimes so uncanny it makes your hair stand on end. A feature of clinical practice since the days of Freud, Ferenczi and Jung, telepathy is currently experiencing a resurgence of interest. This volume provides a comprehensive introduction to contemporary work on this fascinating topic."

Dan Gilhooley, Psy.D., Research Faculty, Boston Graduate School of Psychoanalysis

Telepathy in the Clinical Process

A Century of Psychoanalytic Mystery

Edited by
Richard Reichbart

Routledge
Taylor & Francis Group
LONDON AND NEW YORK

Designed cover image: *Starry Night Over the Rhone*, by Vincent Van Gogh (September 1888). Oil on canvas, 72.5 × 92 cm (28.5 × 36.2 in). Musée d'Orsay, Paris.

First published 2027
by Routledge
4 Park Square, Milton Park, Abingdon, Oxon OX14 4RN

and by Routledge
605 Third Avenue, New York, NY 10158

Routledge is an imprint of the Taylor & Francis Group, an informa business

British Library Cataloguing-in-Publication Data
A catalogue record for this book is available from the British Library

ISBN: 978-1-041-00660-2 (hbk)
ISBN: 978-1-041-00658-9 (pbk)
ISBN: 978-1-003-61104-2 (ebk)

DOI: 10.4324/9781003611042

Typeset in Times New Roman
by Taylor & Francis Books

This book is dedicated to all those psychoanalysts who from the very beginning of psychoanalysis have investigated telepathy in the clinical process.

Contents

Figures

Contributor's Biographies

Richard Reichbart, Ph.D., is a Training and Supervising Analyst and past President (twice) of the Institute for Psychoanalytic Training and Research (IPTAR). He is the author of the book *The Paranormal Surrounds Us: Psychic Phenomena in Literature, Culture and Psychoanalysis* (McFarland, 2019), which features the parapsychological elements in the works of Shakespeare, Joyce, Tolstoy, Foster, Chesterton and Ingmar Bergman; the principles enunciated by Freud with regard to telepathy in the clinical process; and the understanding of parapsychological phenomena in Navajo and other indigeneous cultures. He has published two other books, *The Anatomy of a Psychotic Experiene* (IPBooks, 2021) and *Curious Stories of Diverse Places: The Cod's Earring, the Click of the Reindeer, and Other Adventures and Even Some Poems* (IPBooks, 2019). He was Executive Producer of the video "Black Psychoanalysts Speak" and Co-Producer of the video "Psychoanalysis in El Barrio." He has published 25 psychoanalytic papers and book reviews. He is a member of the Parapsychological Association and the American Psychoanalytic Association (APsaA) and a Fellow of the International Psychoanalytic Association (IPA). He maintains a private practice for children and adults in Ho-Ho-Kus, New Jersey.

Ofra Eshel, Psy.D., is a Training and Supervising Analyst and Senior Faculty member of the Israel Psychoanalytic Society and Institute; fellow, the International psychoanalytic Association (IPA); Honorary Member of the New Center for Psychoanalysis (NCP), Los Angeles, and former vice-president of the International Winnicott Association (IWA). Founder and head of the post-graduate program "Winnicott, Bion, and Independent Psychoanalysis: Radical Breakthroughs" at the advanced studies of the Program of Psychoanalytic Psychotherapy, Faculty of Medicine, Tel-Aviv University. Her papers have been published in psychoanalytic journals and book chapters, translated into ten languages, and presented at national and international conferences across four continents. She has been the recipient of several honors and awards, including visiting scholar at PINC (San Francisco, 2013), visiting lecturer and supervisor at the advanced international training program in

Winnicott's psychoanalysis (Beijing, China, 2018), and Master Class at DeepSprings, (Beijing, China, 2023–2024). She has been honored as the Lecturer of the Psychoanalytic Center of California's 8th Annual Wilfred Bion Conference (Los Angeles, 2018), and the 2021 Robert Stoller Lecture speaker (NCP, Los Angeles), and has been awarded the 2013 Frances Tustin International Memorial Prize and lecture, the 2017 Symonds Prize, and the 2022 Leonard J. Comess Award. In 2012 she was featured in *Globes* (Israel's financial newspaper and magazine) as sixteenth of the 50 most influential women in Israel. She co-edited *Was It or Was It Not? When Shadows of Sexual Abuse Emerge in Psychoanalytic Treatment* (2017) and authored *The Emergence of Analytic Oneness: Into the Heart of Psychoanalysis* (Routledge, 2019), translated into Chinese in 2023. She is in private practice in Tel Aviv, Israel.

Mary Tennes, Ph.D., is a Supervising and Training Analyst and Faculty at the Psychoanalytic Institute of Northern California (PINC). She has taught, presented and published for the last 25 years on the intersection of psychoanalysis and the uncanny, most recently a presentation on Robert Stoller's posthumously published telepathy paper and another titled "Tell All the Truth and Tell It Slant: Psychoanalysis and the Uncanny" to be published soon in *Contemporary Psychoanalysis.* She is in private practice in Oakland, CA.

Janine de Peyer, LCSW-R, is Faculty and Supervisor at the National Institute for the Psychotherapies, New York; the Florida Psychoanalytic Center; and the Stephen Mitchell Relational Study Center. She is Associate Editor with *Psychoanalytic Dialogues*, and has presented internationally on transference-countertransference, eroticism, dissociation, and uncanny communication in the therapeutic dyad. Publications include *Uncanny Communication and the Porous Mind* (Psychoanalytic Dialogues, 2016); *Skating on Thin Ice: Clinical Dilemmas With the Uncanny* (British Psychological Society, Psychotherapy Section Review, 2022); "Telepathic Entanglements: Where are we Today? Commentary on Paper by Claudie Massicotte" (*Psychoanalytic Dialogues*, 2014); and *Unspoken Rhapsody: Female Erotic Countertransference and the Dissociation of Desire, Psychoanalytic Perspectives* (2021). Originally from London, Janine is in private practice in New York City where she integrates EMDR within a relational psychoanalytic framework.

Renaud Evrard is a clinical psychologist, Assistant Professor in Psychology at the University of Lorraine, Nancy, France. He co-founded in 2009, with Thomas Rabeyron, the Center for Information, Research and Counseling on Exceptional Experiences (CIRCEE). He has been president of the Parapsychological Association. He has published "La légende de l'esprit: enquête sur 150 ans de parapsychologie" (Trajectoire, 2016) as well as over 140 journal articles primarily in parapsychology.

Júlia Gyimesi is a Senior Lecturer and Department Head of the Department of Personality and Clinical Psychology at Pázmány Péter Catholic University, Hungary. She is Program Director of the Theoretical Psychoanalysis PhD Program at the University of Péc and a Lecturer of the English-language PhD Program in Psychotherapy Science at the Sigmund Freud Private University in Vienna. She is a historian of psychology with a particular focus on the esoteric antecedents of psychology and has published on the history of animal magnetism, spiritualism, psychical research, early parapsychology, hypnosis, epilepsy, and the Budapest School of psychoanalysis. Currently, she is the board member of the European Society for the Study of Western Esotericism, the European Society for the History of the Human Sciences and the Central and Eastern European Network for the Academic Study of Western Esotericism. Selected articles on the relationship between psychoanalysis and the "occult" include: "Why 'Spiritism'?" *The International Journal of Psychoanalysis* (2016); "Sándor Ferenczi and the Problem of Telepathy," *History of the Human Sciences* (2012); and "The Problem of Demarcation: Psychoanalysis and the Occult," *American Imago* (2009).

Ruth Rosenbaum, Ph.D., L.P., is a faculty member, supervisor and training analyst at NPAP, and a member of the Editorial Board of The Psychoanalytic Review. She also teaches at Columbia University's Teachers College in the graduate Counseling and Clinical Psychology Department. She writes and lectures on the process of change in psychoanalysis, bridging the analytic field with fields such as neuroscience, quantum physics, and studies of psi phenomena. She has presented internationally at scientific conferences on topics such as "Consciousness, Quantum Physics and the Space of Transformation in Psychotherapy." She also lectures on the underlying connection between the long-standing psychoanalytic taboo regarding psi phenomena and the field's lingering avoidance of certain aspects of female sexuality. Publications include: "Exploring the Other Dark Continent: Parallels between Psi Phenomena and the Psychotherapeutic Process," *The Psychoanalytic Review* (2011); "Psychoanalysis, psi phenomena, and spiritual space: Common ground," in *The Oxford Handbook of Psychology and Spirituality* (Oxford University Press, 2012) and the updated edition (2024).

Fonya Helm, Ph.D., ABPP, is a clinical psychologist and psychoanalyst in private practice in Virginia Beach, VA. She is a Training and Supervising Analyst both at the Contemporary Freudian Society and the Institute for Contemporary Psychotherapy and Psychoanalysis. For ten years, she was Chair of the Dynamics of Psychotherapy Training Program at the Washington School of Psychiatry. Publications include: "Book Review of The Paranormal Surrounds Us: Psychic Phenomena in Literature, Culture and Psychoanalysis by Richard Reichbart. *International Journal of Psychoanalysis* (2020); and "Free Association Continues," *Psychoanalytic Inquiry* (2018).

Karen Peoples, Ph.D., is a personal/supervising analyst and faculty at the Psychoanalytic Institute of Northern California and Faculty at the San Francisco Center for Psychoanalysis. She practices in San Francisco and Corte Madera, CA. She has published and presented on numerous analytic topics, including incest and social trauma, uncanny unconscious communication, transcendent and traumatic forms of emptiness, and unconscious bodily communication.

Mikita Brottman, D.Phil., Ph.D., originally from England, is a Professor in the Department of Humanistic Studies at the Maryland Institute of the College of Art in Baltimore. She is a psychoanalyst. She has published 15 books including *Phantoms of the Clinic: From Thought-transference to Projective Identification* (Karnac, 2011) and *Funny Peculiar: Gershon Legman and the Psychopathology of Humor* (Analytic Press, 2004). Her other areas of expertise are non-fiction explorations of crime and criminals, including her book on the experience of teaching a literature course in a prison setting, *The Maximum Security Book Club: Reading Literature in a Men's Prison* (Harper Perennial, 2017), and studies of film.

João Carlos Braga graduated in Medicine at the Federal University of Paraná, Brazil (1966). He was a fellow at Baylor University, Department of Psychiatry, Houston, Texas, (1967). He was Assistant Professor of the Department of Psychiatry and Medical Psychology, Federal University of Paraná (1968–81). He was in private practice in psychiatry and psychotherapy (1968–85) and graduated as Psychoanalyst at Brazilian Psychoanalytic Society of São Paulo (1985). Presently a full member, training and supervising analyst at the Brazilian Psychoanalytic Society of São Paulo, as well as Faculty member. He is founder, training and supervising analyst at Curitiba's Psychoanalytic Group, Brazil. He has been in psychoanalytic practice in Curitiba, Brazil, since 1985. Dr. Braga has around 30 psychoanalytical papers and book chapters published in national and international reviews.

Thomas Rabeyron is a clinical psychologist and a professor of clinical psychology and psychopathology at the university of Lyon at the Centre de Recherche en Psychopathologie et Psychologie Clinique (UR653) and an Honorary Research Fellow at the University of Edinburgh. In 2009, he co-founded the Center for Information, Research and Counseling for Exceptional Experiences (CIRCEE), of which he is director of the counseling service. His research focuses on the clinical aspects of exceptional experiences, neuropsychoanalysis and the evaluation of psychoanalytic psychotherapies. Laureate of the Institut Universitaire de France as a junior member in 2021, he has published 80 scientific papers and two books about clinical psychology (*Psychologie clinique et Psychopathologie*, Armand Colin, 2018) and exceptional experiences (*Clinique des expériences Exceptionnelles*, Dunod, 2020).

Acknowledgements

This collection is possible only because of the determined work of many people. To begin with, I thank those who have contributed the chapters here and who took part in innumerable virtual meetings over three years as well as contributing to the two-day virtual presentation at the New York City-based Institute for Psychoanaltyic Training and Research (IPTAR) on which this book is based. They have joined together from various countries and orientations with a mutual concern and respect for each other; they have all been truly wonderful in their professionalism and their openness, to say nothing of their bravery in publicly pursuing this subject.

In addition, I thank the Institute for Psychoanalytic Training and Research (IPTAR) for mounting the two-day conference, and particularly the chairs of the Program Committee Steven Ellman and Masha Mimram, as well as Aneta Stojnic and Camille Starling-Dade.

Thanks to Routledge which undertook to publish this collection and which has been on the forefront of publishing psychoanalytic books related to telepathy. I am grateful especially to the editor Susannah Frearson who was encouraging from the beginning, to Eleanor Taylor, to Jane Fieldsend for her wonderful competence and of course to Saloni Singhania who shepherded the book through with unwavering attention. In addition, this book would not have been possible without the expertise of Kristopher Spring who edited it with grace and acumen.

On a personal note, I am thankful to the late Jule Eisenbud, my first psychoanalyst, who many years ago in addition to healing me, introduced me to the fields of psychoanalysis and parapsychology. Without him, this collection would never have happened. Last, I am indebted to my companion of 30 plus years, Nansie Ross, who has been patient and loving, making this book possible.

Introduction

Richard Reichbart

On June 1 and 2, 2024, a two-day teleconference was held by the Institute for Psychoanalytic Training and Research, known as IPTAR—a component society of the International Psychoanalytic Association—in New York City. The conference was unusual. First, the subject matter of the conference was striking, reflected in the title of the conference: "A Century of Psychoanalytic Mystery: Telepathy in the Clinical Process." The title was conceived to honor and mark Sigmund Freud's often overlooked 1922 paper, "Dreams and Telepathy," which is one of the four papers he published on telepathy (to say nothing of the numerous letters he wrote about the subject).

The second unusual aspect of the conference was that the presenters (all senior psychoanalytic clinicians as well as a former president of the Parapsychology Association) were from a variety of locations, namely Brazil, France, Hungary, Israel, and the East and West coasts of the United States. Moreover, not only were the presenters from a variety of locations, they favored a variety of psychoanalytic orientations, from contemporary Freudian to Bionian to Winnicottian to Relational—each presenter, despite theoretical differences, nonetheless speaking on the same subject: telepathy in the clinical process.

Out of this conference comes the book before you, of the same title. The chapters offered here are similar to the conference presentations, although some have been further elaborated. But before going further, let me pose some questions that will undoubtedly come to mind. First, how did these psychoanalysts—or let me change the way I am stating this: how did *we* psychoanalysts from such different venues and from such different orientation—manage to get together for a conference on telepathy in the psychoanalytic process in the first place? And why telepathy? And why this resulting book?

Telepathy may seem strange to some, but the fact is that the study of it in the clinical process has been in existence since the very beginning of psychoanalysis. And although it has been explored by psychoanalysts from Freud on, as a subject it has too often been sidelined, denied, forgotten, misunderstood, minimized, and ridiculed despite the fact that the clinical data about it within psychoanalysis have been voluminous. Further, telepathy in

DOI: 10.4324/9781003611042-1

psychoanalytic treatment has often proved crucial to understanding the patient and the patient's relationship to the psychoanalyst, and it has often played a transformative role in transference and countertransference that exists between patient and analyst. In fact, as you will see from the chapters that follow, it has sometimes been crucial to the curative process in moving and intriguing ways.

Each of the presenters of the conference, now authors in this book, firmly believes in telepathy's importance to psychoanalytic treatment, based on our own (often surprising) experiences of it in clinical process. Over recent years, each of us has written and published peer-reviewed articles or books on telepathy, and many of us have presented about it internationally. Our backgrounds and publications concerning telepathy in psychoanalysis are compiled in the author biographies at the beginning of this book.

Not only do we each present here about telepathy in clinical practice, but we present about the history of telepathy in psychoanalysis: the role it played from the very start with Freud, Ferenczi, and Jung. In addition, you will learn the extent to which Freud, despite his ambivalence and despite the efforts of Ernest Jones to discourage him, actually enunciated principles on how to handle telepathy in treatment. Because this aspect of psychoanalytic treatment is so often ignored or subsumed in ways that deny its essential existence under such terms as "unconscious communication," I am taking the liberty of listing only some of the analysts who have accepted and written on this in the past: Freud, Ferenczi, Jung, Balint, Gillespie (former president of the International Psychoanalytic Association), Dorothy Burlingham, Hollos, Hitschmann, Fodor, Eisenbud, Ehrenwald, Greenson, Elizabeth Lloyd Mayer, Pederson-Krag, Roheim, Helene Deutsch, Stoller, Ullman, Eduardo Weiss, and Servadio.

In fact, publications on telepathy by many of these listed psychoanalysts appeared in a long-ago seminal collection edited by George Devereux, *Psychoanalysis and the Occult* (1953). At that time, that is in the 1950s–1960s, there was an upsurge of interest in telepathy and precognition in psychoanalysis, featuring the work of the psychoanalysts Eisenbud, Ehrenwald, Ullman, Fodor, and Servadio, and encouraged in New York City by the American Society for Psychical Research (today more or less moribund) and the psychic Elleen Garrett's Parapsychology Foundation. But that interest was rapidly squelched by established psychoanalysis. For example, the doyen of the New York Psychoanalytic Institute, Charles Brenner in 1987 claiined that as a result of an article he published thirty yers previously (1957) he had singlehandedly succeeded in preventing any further publication in established psychoanalytic journals of articles on telepathy, contending that he at least knew what was "real." The pages of established journals ceased carrying such articles (despite the fact that the study of telepathy had been featured early on in the establishment of psychoanalysis), and those analysts listed above who explored the subject have since passed.

Today, 70 years later, we analysts have taken up the effort to explore telepathy in clinical process once again and hope that this volume can be a worthy follow-up to Devereux's 1953 collection. Much of what we present here is not new, for periodically this type of data is "rediscovered." But perhaps it will have more cogency today, when transference and countertransference have gained ascendance. Today, in addition to this data, we present various theoretical ideas about why and how telepathy takes place in treatment. Some of these ideas are shared among the analysts writing here, but others are a source of disagreement, which we also explore. More than anything else, however, we hope to intrigue and even startle the reader about what can happen in clinical process, as Freud himself was intrigued and startled 100 years ago.

How did we as psychoanalysts happen to get together about telepathy? In 2019, I published *The Paranormal Surrounds Us: Psychic Phenomena in Literature, Culture and Psychoanalysis*, which deals not only with telepathy, but with other psychic phenomena. I had come to explore psychic phenomena because of my first analysis with Jule Eisenbud, one of the most prominent psychoanalysts publishing in this area who was also a parapsychologist. Among other things, my book compiled work from many years ago that I had published in the parapsychological *Journal of the American Society for Psychical Research*, including a study of the psychic in Navajo Indian culture (where I had worked as a legal services attorney) as well as studies of great Western literature, such as Tolstoy's *Anna Karenina* and Foster's *A Passage to India*, and then years later for my book, Shakespeare's *Hamlet*, Joyce's *Ulysses*, and G. K. Chesterton's play *Magic*, which Ingmar Bergman adapted in his film *The Magician*. I contended that intuitively these great writers understood and accurately depicted the workings of psychic phenomena, particularly telepathy.

In addition, I wrote about telepathy in psychoanalysis and was aware of the striking work of the psychoanalysts here, many of whom I cited in my paranormal book—certainly the work of Ofra Eshel from Israel; Janine de Peyer's publications; the work of Ruth Rosenbaum from NPAP, who had been a friend for years; Julia Gyimesi, whose work in Hungary I admired from afar; and Fonya Helm, who with Maureen Kelly has held a discussion group on Altered States at the annual American Psychoanalytic Association conference in New York, where they invited me to speak in 2020. I also was aware of the work of Mikita Brottman, whose wonderful book *Phantoms of the Clinic* was published in 2011, which among other things attempted to resurrect the work of the psychoanalyst/parapsychologist Jule Eisenbud.

But then, to my complete surprise, Thomas Rabeyron, Evrard Renaud, and Claudie Massicote from France—I had never heard of Thomas or Evrard—managed to get published in the June 2021 *Journal of the American Psychoanalytic Association* (*JAPA*) the paper "Psychoanalysis in the Telepathic Process"—a remarkable achievement, given *JAPA*'s contemporary reluctance to publish on psychic phenomena—and an article I highly recommend. (Both Evrard and Thomas contributed to the IPTAR program and now to this book.) I used their article as a springboard to contact all the psychoanalysts here and for all of us to get together by Zoom. Everyone agreed. Ofra Eshel then brought in Mary Tennes and Karen Peoples from the West coast of the United States (as opposed to the East coast, where the rest of the United States contingent was from) and eventually the Bionian analyst Joao Braga from Brazil. We met once every month or so over three years, sharing our experiences, many of which were deeply personal. Finally, we decided to present together at the IPTAR virtual conference, and subsequently it became apparent to us that we had the makings of a book.

Routledge—which to its credit had recently published two books by the Italian psychoanalyst Maria Pierri, *Occultism and the Origins of Psychoanalysis: Freud, Ferenczi and the Challenge of Thought Transference* (2018) and *Sigmund Freud and the Forsyth Case: Coincidences and Thought-Transmission in Psychoanalysis* (2022), placing Routledge at the forefront of the effort to focus on telepathy and psychoanalysis—readily agreed to publish this book.

So here it is. We believe the material presented here is not only intriguing, but it is fundamental and important to the clinical process. It provides an avenue, often of intimacy between patient and psychoanalyst, that can lead to dynamic change. And in addition, in some but not all of these chapters, you will discover material that leads outside the clinical process to a seemingly wider psychic world of which telepathy hints.

References

Brenner, C. (1987). Notes on psychoanalysis by a participant observer: A personal chronical. *Journal of the American Psychoanalytic Association*, 39, 539–555.

Brottman, M. (2011). *Phantoms of the Clinic: From thought-transference to projective identification*. Karnac.

Devereux, G. (Ed.) (1953). *Psychoanalysis and the occult*. International Universities Press.

Freud, S. (1922). Dreams and telepathy. In J. Strachey (Ed. & Trans.), *The standard edition of the complete psychological works of Sigmund Freud* (Vol. 18, pp. 195–220). Hogarth Press.

Pierri, M. (2018). *Occultism and the origins of psychoanalysis: Freud, Ferenczi and the challenge of thought transference* (A. Elgar, Trans.). Routledge.

Pierri, M. (2022). *Sigmund Freud and the Forsyth case: Coincidences and thought-transmission in psychoanalysis* (A. Elgar, Trans.). Routledge.

Rabeyron, T., Evrard, R., & Massicotte, C. (2021). Psychoanalysis and the telepathic process. *Journal of the American Psychoanalytic Association*, 69, 535–571.

Reichbart, R. (2019). *The paranormal surrounds us: Psychic phenomena in literature, culture and psychoanalysis.* McFarland.

Chapter 1

Where Are You, My Beloved?

On Absence, Loss, and the Enigma of Telepathic Dreams

Ofra Eshel

Ofra Eshel, Ph.D., the prominent Israeli psychoanalyst whose work is inspired by Freud, Winnicott, and Bion, and whose 2019 book The Emergence of Analytic Oneness: Into the Heart of Psychoanalysis, *speaks to patient–analyst interconnectedness and the importance of the analyst giving herself over to the patient's experiential world, opens this collection with an article that reveals unexpected telepathic communication between her and certain patients. She presents analytic encounters over the years with the telepathic dreams of five patients—dreams involving precise details of time, place, sensory impressions, and experiential states that Ofra was in at the time which the patient could not have known through ordinary sensory perception. The mother of each of these patients in early childhood was emotionally absent, although physically present. This resulted for the patient in a fixation on a nonverbal, archaic mode of communication, that is unconscious telepathy. The patient's telepathy in her dreams served as a search engine to find the analyst when the analyst also was suddenly emotionally absent, and thus to halt the process of abandonment and prevent a collapse into the despair of the early traumatization.*

* * * *

Dream telepathy (especially patients' telepathic dreams), and related telepathic phenomena in the psychoanalytic context, have been a highly controversial, disturbing "foreign body" ever since telepathy was introduced into psychoanalysis by Freud in 1921.

In Laplanche and Pontalis's dictionary *The Language of Psychoanalysis* (1988), there is no mention of telepathy or related phenomena in the psychoanalytic context. Yet, over the years, sporadic psychoanalytic writings on possibly telepathic experiences, and particularly patients' telepathic dreams, have accumulated and amounted to a body of clinical observations that deserve serious consideration. However, this was met with trepidation, from Freud's first article on this subject (written in 1921 but only published posthumously 20 years later) to Stoller's paper "Telepathic Dreams?", written in 1973 but published posthumously 28 years later by Mayer (2001). Even this cursory information brings us directly and intriguingly into the heart of the

DOI: 10.4324/9781003611042-2

controversy over and resistance to the idea of telepathy, which forced itself like "a foreign body" into psychoanalysis (Derrida, 1988; Freud, 1933; Major & Miller, 1981; Torok, 1986)—"a crypt that threw psychoanalysis, Freud included, into confusion ever since the 1920s" (Torok, 1986, p. 96); indeed, a disturbing, "impossible" topic in "the impossible profession" (to use Freud's 1937 locution). Delving into the profound mystery of telepathy in psychoanalysis is thought-provoking and complex, fraught with astonishment and discomfort often verging on a deeper trepidation (Eshel, 2006, 2019a, 2019b). Yet, I think that we are called to engage with it, as expressed powerfully by Freud's groundbreaking words and Derrida's response to this calling:

> It is a very remarkable thing that the *Ucs.* of one human being can react upon that of another, without passing through the *Cs.* This deserves closer investigation ... but, descriptively speaking, the fact is incontestable.
>
> Freud (1915, p. 194)

> If only one accustoms oneself to the idea of telepathy, one can accomplish a great deal with it—for the time being, it is true, only in imagination ... All this is still uncertain and full of unsolved riddles; but there is no reason to be frightened by it.
>
> Freud (1933, p. 55)

> So, touch with both ends at once, touch in the area where science and so-called technical objectivity are now taking hold of it instead of resisting it as they used to ... touch in the area of our immediate apprehensions, our pathies, our receptions, our apprehensions because we are letting ourselves be approached without taking or comprehending anything and because we are afraid.
>
> Derrida (1988, p. 13)

In the present chapter, I will focus on and explore the profound enigma of patients' telepathic dreams from *my own analytic experiences* with them. But, for me, this is a crucial point. For it was only when I was faced in my practice with telepathic occurrences—unusual, surprising, rare, and inexplicable—that my interest in them and my search for an explanation evolved. There were five "telepathic" dreams by five patients over my 35 years of clinical experience—dreams that "knew" or occurred in the very place, time, and experiential state that I was in then. They made it absolutely necessary for me to presume the possibility of information-transfer between patient and analyst in another, different way, one that goes beyond ordinary senses and speech. In this way, I arrived at telepathy (from the Greek: *tele*—far, distant + *pathos*—suffering, intense feeling), a term coined by the English psychologist Frederic Myers in 1882 to "cover all cases of impression received at a distance without the normal operation of the recognized sense organs" (Royle, 1991).

This process evolved over time: The first two "telepathic" dreams took me by surprise when my patients recounted them (several years apart), but I then pushed them to some remote corner of my mind. My approach changed only when such dreams recurred three more times over the years, with other patients. These—starting from the third dream that I will present here in detail—remained in my thoughts, seeking to be resolved.

"Allow ourselves to be touched, wounded, and demolished in our own *being* … in order to try to approach what is radically other" (Pontalis, 2003, p. 11). I believe that, over time, I allowed my patients' telepathic dreams to touch and strike me. I let the feelings of incomprehension and discomfort invoked by these dreams linger in my thoughts, and I tried to psychoanalytically fathom their meaning, essence, and enigmatic emergence in the analytic process. It also led me to the intriguing psychoanalytic literature written over the years on the vicissitudes of the psychoanalytic encounter with telepathic dreams (Devereux, 1953; Eshel, 2006, 2019a).

I will now describe this third encounter with my patients' telepathic dreams, and then the understanding that has crystallized in me over the years, which has found an echo and backing in the psychoanalytic literature.

Case Illustration: "You Alone Knew How to Wait/Search"

Background

Effie (Efrat) came to analysis because of feeling increasingly unreal and detached from her husband, her four-year-old daughter, and her immediate environment, feelings unrelated to external circumstances. She would later add that these feelings had perhaps intensified since her daughter was about six months old.

At the beginning of analysis, Effie recounted the dramatic story of her early childhood. Both her mother and maternal grandmother were Holocaust survivors. They had fled with a neighbor's family from their home in Poland to Russia. Her mother's husband of barely a year, and her mother's father, along with the rest of the family, were due to join them a few days later, but they were caught and sent to concentration camps, where they perished.

During the war, Effie's mother and grandmother survived extreme hardship, hunger, and mortal terror. At the end of the war, they immigrated to Israel and attempted to rebuild their lives. Not a single relative, close or distant, had survived. Despite exhaustive efforts, they found no one who could provide additional information about what had happened to the rest of the family. They were totally alone; even the neighbor's family, with whom they had escaped, had immigrated to a different country.

Effie's mother found work, and a few years later remarried and had two daughters, of which Effie was the younger. During that period, with the help of her mother who lived in close proximity, she stopped working and began studying in university.

Then, a crucial, devastating event occurred in their lives, an event about which Effie had only partial knowledge. When she was about ten months old, her mother's first husband suddenly reappeared. Effie did not know how he had found her mother, whether and how many times they had met, or whether they had only communicated by letters or phone. Apparently, they did meet. He too had remarried and had two young children, although Effie did not know who had remarried first; it seems they had remarried about the same time. He reappeared and then disappeared forever; Effie did not know whether he lived in some distant part of Israel or abroad. But he was never seen or heard from again. She did not know whether this had been a joint decision.

Effie's mother then withdrew and shut herself in her room. She would not respond, would not relate, refused to see anybody. Her mother (Effie's grandmother) was called upon to help out and moved in with the family. She was a caring, devoted woman who mainly attended to meals and the family's other basic needs. Only two sounds cut through the silence in the house: the radio, which all day long and most of the night was tuned to the program *Searching for Lost Relatives*, and the song "Wait for Me and I'll Come Back," which Effie's mother listened to over and over on the record player, alone in her closed room. Effie's father would return from work and sit on the balcony, sucking at his pipe in silence and staring out into the garden; at first, he slept in the sitting room and later the balcony was enclosed so he could sleep there.

After about ten months, Effie's mother came out of her room and switched off the record player, and the song was no longer played. She went back to university, immersed herself in her studies, made up the year she had missed, continued studying and, in time, carved out an impressive academic career in her field. Effie's grandmother, replaced by a nanny, returned to her own home but continued to be actively involved in their lives at home. The radio continued to broadcast *Searching for Lost Relatives*, but at a reduced volume, and only when Effie's mother or grandmother were home; they both continued to listen to it anxiously. Only once a year, every year, from the eve of Holocaust Remembrance Day to its end the following evening, would Effie's mother light a memorial candle and play the record once again in her room, and the sounds of the song "Wait for Me and I'll Come Back," by now scratched and worn, would reverberate relentlessly throughout the house, all that night and day. The candle burned, the song played, and Effie's mother remained shut in her room, every year on that day. When Effie quoted me the words of this familiar old song, they suddenly seemed so harsh, poignant, and painful to me:

> Wait for me and I'll come back!
> Just you truly wait,
> Wait when Autumn's dreary rains
> Wait when snow is falling fast,
> Wait when summer's hot,
> Wait when yesterdays are past,

Others are forgot.
Wait though from that far-off place
No letters come to you.
Wait when others cease to wait,
All who waited too.
Wait for me and I'll come back! …
Even when my dearest ones
Say that I am lost
Even when my friends give up …
Wait, don't give up hope.

Wait for me and I'll come back,
Defying every death!
"What a bit of luck!" they'll say,
Those that did not wait.
They will never understand
How amidst the strife,
By your waiting for me, dear
You have saved my life.
How I made it, we shall know,
Only I and you.
You alone knew how to *search*
As no other knew.
(Konstantin Simonov, 1941)

"You alone knew how to *search* as no other knew," Effie recited the last line. "You alone knew how to *wait*," I corrected the word, unable now to recall if silently or out loud, and not yet knowing that she had thus conveyed to me, without my understanding, the very heart of the telepathic occurrence.

Apparently, after that very difficult year, family life in Effie's home returned to normal. They talked little of feelings—"but maybe it was also like that before the crisis," said Effie. It was only years later, in late adolescence, that Effie learned from her sister and an elderly relative on her father's side about "the hard year." It began with the relative's comment that Holocaust Remembrance Day was so sad in their house, not just because their grandfather and the rest of the family had perished, but also because of "that man." Effie's efforts to find out more details were in vain; her sister and the elderly relative knew little. Her sister was four years older but had been only a young child at the time. Effie had never dared ask her mother and father, and they themselves never talked about it, while her grandmother refused to speak of those "old, sad matters." "My little girl" ("*Mein kind,*" she would say in Yiddish), "we went through so many terrible things, you know, thank God, we got through it all, there's no point in talking about it, leave it alone, it's over and done with, everything is fine," she would say over and over, kindly but firmly, each time Effie broached the subject, and then fall silent or change the subject.

"Everything was fine" in Effie's life too. She did well in school, went on to university, married an older man, and started a family; but the feeling of meaninglessness in her life grew ever stronger. Her grandmother died and then her father, and she "felt nothing." "I began to feel that my fate would be like that of Hannah in *My Michael* by the Israeli writer Amos Oz," she said (The book tells of 30-year-old Hannah's growing withdrawal from her husband Michael and her young child, into a private, disconnected fantasy world). Effie felt that the book's opening sentences very closely related to her:

> I am writing this because people I loved have died. I am writing this because when I was a child I was full of the power of loving, and now that power of loving is dying. *I do not want to die.*
>
> (1972, p. 1, Effie's emphasis)

And so, she came to analysis. She came to me because she had heard that my approach was Winnicottian.

The Dream

During the first year of analysis (of four times a week, on the couch), Effie conveyed pervasive feelings of not belonging and heaviness, and particularly had difficulty talking. "Basically, I never talked. I don't really know how to talk about feelings," she said. "I know how to organize, put all sorts of things in order and then … a vacuum." She felt "so heavy, not understood, not belonging, not connected to anybody. Once I had such a need to belong, but I got stuck somewhere in the middle." I felt her agonizing loneliness. She was very conscientious about coming to analysis, rarely missing a session or arriving late, but feared and blocked all feelings of connection, neediness, and dependence. In the sessions, I often felt that I had to hold her firmly lest she slip away through the empty spaces in her words. Yet, as the year drew to a close, a gradual, subtle shift seemed to occur in her tone of voice and in her intense feelings of isolation and desperateness.

The dream I describe was recounted at the beginning of the second year of analysis, on a Thursday, the third session of the week (we had no sessions on Wednesdays).

Effie began by saying she was "feeling better now." She was silent for a moment, then continued that she was "coming back" from being detached; she had had two difficult days, everyone said she had been completely detached. She fell silent, then went on. Her husband talked to her, but she couldn't hear. It seemed to her that I too had been detached on Tuesday, maybe also on Monday. She was silent again. I asked her whether she thought that her being detached was related to my being detached. She said haltingly, "My body feels weightless. Floating. Not a pleasant feeling. Frightening." She was speaking with great difficulty. I said, "Effie, you were talking about my detachment and you became detached. Come back down to me and tell me what's happening." She slowly began to say that she had slept poorly the previous two nights, on Tuesday and Wednesday. Last night, she awoke very early and remembered a dream, which she then recounted. (As is my habit, I wrote the dream down as she told it, and it is presented here verbatim.)

> What I remember is that I am in a different country, hurrying to the place where my father is buried, which I know is about to close at four o'clock. I manage to get there a few minutes before, go into some sort of entrance hall and from there I see that the gate I have to go through is closing. It's no longer possible to go in. I try to persuade the gatekeeper to let me in. I explain to him that I've come from a different place, far away, and I've already come in, and it's very important for me to come in because not being there, and he lets me in. And then I go into some sort of room, with a picture of my father hanging on the left, and next to it several other pictures. Like below the wall, underneath the floor, that is actually where my father is buried, it's not clear to me whether alone or with other people. I don't remember. It's as if the whole way he's buried is so different. And it's as if also in the dream I feel myself different. The entire time I'm someone else, I think. I'm not alone, I think.

She was silent and then continued,

> I usually don't manage to explain how important things are for me. I don't feel good about that. I feel myself not understood. That's how it feels to me—people don't understand me, then I become very tense, and then everything gets messed up. But here I said, "*I've already come in. I've come from far away, it's very important for me to go in, let me come in,*" and he lets me in. And my father's picture. A beautiful picture. He's smiling. There's a feeling of longing. That's something very new, this dream. Up to now my experience with dreams was that they confirm things I've already experienced in life, confirming them through a different medium.

I listened in astonishment to the dream and to the things she said. She dreamed the dream on Wednesday night, and Wednesday afternoon I had attended a memorial service in the cemetery for my own father that began at four o'clock. And I had felt intense longing. I had been very attached to my father, and, around the time of the memorial service this year, due to certain family issues, I had especially missed him. I am certain that Effie had no way of knowing where I had been that day. I also realized that I had indeed been detached on Tuesday, and perhaps also on Monday, without being aware of it.

What encounter with me was Effie struggling for beyond the disconnection, beyond the closed gate, in spite of death and deadness? It was as if she had entered my mind, had been in a place and time I had been in, inside the longing I had felt. "I've come from a *different place, far away*, and I've already come in, and it's very important for me to come in because not being there," she had said to the gatekeeper, and he let her in. Who was it that was "not there"—her, me? The old, deep scar of absence had suddenly reopened, speaking, pleading.

I deliberated whether to tell her all this; I asked questions about the dream and more was said, mostly about her parents, especially her father's years-long emotional distance from her world. Finally, about ten minutes before the end of the session, I decided to tell her, since so much had not been told to her in her life and had not been talked about with her. I said, "You know, Effie, yesterday I was really in the cemetery for my father's memorial service, at four in the afternoon. And maybe this affected my being detached and your being detached and your dream."

She remained silent until the end of the session and then said, "It is amazing and frightening how much things that happen to you affect me. Do you understand the enormousness of your responsibility?"

"Cry Open in a Forest of Frost, in a Dawn of Cornflowers": The Telepathic Dream between Absence and Complete Loss

In four decades of clinical work, I encountered five telepathic dreams. These five dreams were sporadic occurrences over the years. Yet they always appeared at emotionally charged, significant moments in *my* life, and involved the precise details of time, place, sensory impressions, and experiential states that I was in at that time—dumbfounding *informational* details, not merely experiential–emotional details—that the patients could not have known through ordinary sensory perception and communication. All were connected to matters of life and death (in this order): a young female patient's dream in which *I was telling her that I was pregnant*, which she dreamed on the very day I found out that I was pregnant (with my eldest daughter); a dream of a male patient who "knew" I had miscarried (a different pregnancy five years later) when I cancelled the sessions on those days; Effie's dream on the night of the memorial service for my father, which was where I was at—in place, hour, and emotional state—on the same day; a detailed cemetery dream by a male patient during the week that both my in-laws died within two days of each other; and a dream about a dying woman that a female patient dreamed three days before my mother's death—during a period when I would leave my mother's deathbed to carry on my analytic work—which depicted very specific details of the situation with my mother on those days, with dumbfounding precision.

All the telepathic elements were unique to these particular dreams and did not recur in these patients' other dreams (see also Stoller, in Mayer, 2001; Ullman, 2003). The first patient was in psychotherapy, and the other four in analysis; the latter dreams were equally divided between men and women.

The explanations of telepathic dreams during treatment in the psychoanalytic literature stem from factors related to the traumatic childhood circumstances of these patients; the ensuing nonverbal, archaic mode of communication, heightened in critical, emotionally laden moments; and the analyst's role in provoking telepathic dreams. In my effort to unravel and understand these enigmatic, abstruse phenomena, a specific set of experiences took on primary importance, combining these three contributing factors: Each of these patients, during *early childhood* (aged a few months to almost two years), had *a mother who was absent, mostly absent-within-absence,* that is, a mother physically present yet emotionally absent from her child's early life, often due to the absence of a significant figure in her own life. In my case examples, it was the absence of the husband–father (except for Effie's special story)—one case due to sudden death, and the others due to a temporary, but prolonged (over six months) absence of the husband–father. In most of the cases, the mother's experiences of absence and separation were intensified by an earlier absence of one or both of *her* parents (due to the Holocaust, lengthy separation, or death).

Thus, the silenced cry of this abrupt and critical early catastrophic trauma resides in a world of primal attachment, in a nonverbal or pre-verbal period, with an ensuing fixation on an archaic mode of communication.

Winnicott (1971), in a memorable passage, describes the formation of x + y + z degree of mother's deprivation:

> The feeling of the mother's existence lasts x minutes. If the mother is away more than x minutes … the baby is distressed, but this distress is soon *mended* because the mother returns in x + y minutes. In x + y minutes the baby has not become altered. But in x + y + z minutes the baby has become *traumatized.* In x + y + z minutes the mother's return does not mend the baby's altered state. Trauma implies that the baby has experienced a break in life's continuity, so that primitive defenses now become organized to defend against a repetition of "unthinkable anxiety" or a return of the acute confusional state that belongs to disintegration of nascent ego structure.
>
> We must assume that the vast majority of babies never experience the x + y + z quantity of deprivation. This means that the majority of children do not carry around with them for life the knowledge from experience of having been mad. Madness here simply means a *break-up* of whatever may exist at the time of a *personal continuity of existence.* After "recovery" from x + y + z deprivation the baby has to start again permanently deprived of the root which could provide *continuity with the personal beginning.*
>
> (pp. 114–155, italics in original)

I would say that the mother who is absent-within-absence creates the $x + y + z$ degree of deprivation/absence, or this is even a case of *double absence*—z^2—which is imprinted in the nascent self and in baby's inchoate relating to others.

Balint (1955) relates telepathic dreams to a patient "in a state of intense positive dependent transference, which however was not fully appreciated and understood by the analyst" (p. 32). But I have found that these patients, because of their early traumatic history, defend themselves against strong and endangering feelings of dependence and becoming attached. Thus, in the treatment process, they struggle to block dependence and will not allow themselves (and the analyst) to feel their deep regressive yearning for the analyst, except in a buried, hidden way. This abruptly changes when, within this intricate situation, the analyst suddenly becomes emotionally (and sometimes also physically) *absent* because his or her attention is significantly diverted to other matters, often to absence in the analyst's own world. Under such circumstances, the patient's dread of reliving the deeply annihilating traumatic absence, the breaking of personal continuity of existence, now bursts forth—never, never again to return to such devastating absence and abandonment, to that maddening, unbearable loss of the early mother.

The telepathic dream is created in *the gap between absence and annihilating loss*, between separation and all-out complete loss; it forms *a search engine to seek and find the analyst, in order to halt the process of abandonment and prevent a return and collapse into the depths of despair of the early catastrophic traumatization*.

Indeed, if tele-pathy is "suffering at a distance" (Greek: *pathos* + *tele*), the *suffering because of distance, suffering over distance* achieves its critical potential here. The telepathic dream ushers us into the very heart of pathos—the suffering, the intense feeling; the patient's pathos, the analyst's pathos. For whose pathos is it? Whose dream? The dreaming patient clings to the analyst *beyond the boundaries of separateness, separation, time, space, and known processes of sensory perception* in a way that is hitherto not scientifically explicable, yet it occurs. The patient manages to enter the analyst's mind and the analyst's private affairs, experiences, absence—but not fully; that is, in a necessary, uncanny way, to telepathically perceive the most salient physical and emotionally charged details, which the ordinary senses fail to provide. Yet not fully.

"*The gate … is closing. It's no longer possible to go in. I try to persuade the gatekeeper to let me in*," said Effie in her dream. Only on rereading these dream words lately, I realized with astonishment how similar they are to the deeply pleading words and the sense of urgency that imbues the final prayer of the Holy Day of Atonement [at-one-ment], the prayer that forms the emotional climax of the pleas that resonate throughout the day: "Open the gate for us at this time when the gate closes, for the day is fading away" (*Neilah*, The Closing of the Gate).

"*I explain to him that I've come from a different place, far away, and I've already come in, and it is very important for me to come in because not being there. And the gatekeeper lets me in*," Effie continued in her dream. On those particular days, she detached herself from her real world and reached me, while I was in a different, emotionally laden, distant place. "*And it's as if in the dream I feel myself different. The entire time I'm someone else, I think. I'm not alone, I think*" [verbatim].

It can be said that the telepathic dream actualizes the possibility of primary, unmediated patient–analyst interconnectedness or analytic oneness in the deepest sense, revealing its power and radical quality:

> Telepathy [is not] an actual transmission of sensory perceptions or of cognitive material from one person to another … We must assume that every telepathic incident involves the temporary fusion of two emotionally linked individuals into one functional unit, re-establishing for a fleeting moment the original mother–child unit as it existed at an early developmental stage.
>
> Ehrenwald (1960, p. 53)

At the same time, it still implies, in its very name and quality, the ultimately irreducible, irremediable distance between two people.

In the telepathic dream, the patient's reach exceeds his or her personal boundaries, turns into a paranormal mode of seeking and receiving information, and reaches-grips-holds onto the analyst—"a psychic prothesis, a stretched-out arm, which reaches out mystically towards that which is far off and cannot be approached in actuality by physical means" (Hitschmann, 1924, p. 438).

Thus, the telepathic dream breaks through the emotional absence and brings the analyst back to the patient, even when it does not make the analyst poignantly aware of his or her emotional absence and the patient's suffering, as Balint (1955) emphatically maintains. And, at its best, the telepathic dream creates *a moment of bare at-one-ness* of patient and analyst (at-one with the other and within oneself), while facing their intense and enigmatic inner interconnection that has now been exposed—thus creating a new observation, a new understanding, a *new possibility.*

Should the analyst—the only one who knows about the telepathic occurrence—tell the patient about it? Opinions are divided on such issues as clinical caution, the analyst's anonymity versus disclosure, and the authenticity of patient–analyst dialogue. Thus, Ehrenwald cautioned analysts not to tell patients until a later stage of analysis, when they would be capable of dealing with the burden of such involvement, while at that time Eisenbud (1946) maintained that, when analysts are careful, gentle, and wise in their handling of telepathic experiences, they can bring about most helpful and meaningful results. Considering these different approaches, Shainberg (1976) writes of his fear that his patient might be scared by the realization of the extent of his involvement with his analyst and chose to avoid risk by not telling the patient. Conversely, Mayer (2001) is resolute about the importance of expanding the ability of patient and analyst alike to examine *all* aspects of what the patient knows about the analyst within the analytic intersubjective relationship, including anomalous telepathic knowledge. She sees this as important both in terms of the psychoanalytic situation and clinical psychoanalytic thinking.

Undoubtedly, this is a sensitive, daring, self-revealing moment, which, at times, is no less difficult and delicate for the analyst than it is for the patient. But I feel that it is a meaningful, authentic and unique (intrapsychic and interpersonal) moment, which allows analyst and patient a different kind of exchange—groping and evolving—while facing their intense and enigmatic unconscious interconnection that has now been exposed. It is a powerful moment of connection that both comes to life and is deepened by this exchange. As Derrida (1988) writes so evocatively:

> You say "It was me," with a gentle and terrible decision ... You say "me" the unique addressee and everything starts between us. Starting out from nothing, from no history ... (committing yourself to it even for eternity) ... you gather it together without reducing it, without harming it, you let it live and everything starts between us, from you, and what you there give by receiving. Others would conclude: a letter thus finds its addressee, him or her. No, one cannot say of the addressee that s/he exists before the letter'[s arrival].
>
> Derrida (1988, p. 6)

In concluding, I find that this account did not take me into the domain of occultism, but rather into *the occult of psychoanalysis and the psychoanalytic process.* It ushered me into the heart of the unfathomable *depth, intensity, and mystery* of the human psyche and its struggle to survive traumatization and retraumatization, and particularly of patient–analyst unconscious quantum interconnectedness[1] in the psychoanalytic situation and its "impossible" extremes, defying space, time, and personal boundaries.

Note

1 I have also called this process in its extreme singularity "quantum interconnectedness" (from physicist David Bohm's 1980 phrase "the quantum interconnectedness of distant systems"), in order to convey the profound implications of this quantum-like psychoanalytic quality of experience (Eshel, 2019a).

References

Balint, M. (1955). Notes on parapsychology and parapsychological healing. *International Journal of Psychoanalysis*, 36, 31–35.

Bohm, D. (1980). *Wholeness and the implicate order.* Routledge.

Derrida, J. (1988). Telepathy (N. Royle, Trans.). *Oxford Literary Review*, 10, 3–41.

Devereux, G. (Ed.). (1953). *Psychoanalysis and the occult.* International Universities Press.

Ehrenwald, J. (1960). Schizophrenia, neurotic compliance, and the psi hypothesis. *Psychoanalytic Review*, 47, 43–54.

Eisenbud, J. (1946). Telepathy and problems of psychoanalysis. *Psychoanalytic Quarterly*, 15, 32–87.

Eshel, O. (2006). Where are you, my beloved? *International Journal of Psychoanalysis*, 87, 1603–1627.

Eshel, O. (2019a). *The emergence of analytic oneness: Into the heart of psychoanalysis.* Routledge.
Eshel, O. (2019b). Would clinical psychoanalysis shy away from delving further into the unknown? On the mystery of telepathic dreams. *International Journal of Psychoanalysis*, 100, 608–610.
Freud, S. (1915). The unconscious. In J. Strachey (Ed. & Trans.), *The standard edition of the complete psychological works of Sigmund Freud* (Vol. 14, pp. 159–216). Hogarth Press.
Freud, S. (1921). Psychoanalysis and telepathy. In J. Strachey (Ed. & Trans.), *The standard edition of the complete psychological works of Sigmund Freud* (Vol. 18, pp. 177–193). Hogarth Press.
Freud, S. (1933). Dreams and occultism. In J. Strachey (Ed. & Trans.), *The standard edition of the complete psychological works of Sigmund Freud* (Vol. 22, pp. 31–56). Hogarth Press.
Freud, S. (1937). Analysis terminable and interminable. In J. Strachey (Ed. & Trans.), *The standard edition of the complete psychological works of Sigmund Freud* (Vol. 23, pp. 216–253). Hogarth Press.
Hitschmann, E. (1924). Telepathy and psychoanalysis. *International Journal of Psychoanalysis*, 5, 425–439.
Laplance, J., & Pontalis, J.-B. (1988). *The language of psychoanalysis.* Routledge.
Major, R., & Miller, P. (1981). Empathy, antipathy and telepathy in the analytic process. *Psychoanalytic Inquiry*, 1, 449–470.
Mayer, E. L. (2001). On "Telepathic dreams?": An unpublished paper by Robert J. Stoller. *Journal of the American Psychoanalytic Association*, 49, 629–657.
Oz, A. (1972). *My Michael* (N. de Lange, Trans.). Chatto & Windus.
Pontalis, J.-B. (2003). *Windows* (A. Quinney, Trans.). University of Nebraska Press.
Royle, N. (1991). *Telepathy and literature: Essays on the leading mind.* Blackwell.
Shainberg, D. (1976). Telepathy in psychoanalysis: An instance. *American Journal of Psychotherapy*, 30, 463–472.
Simonov, K.(1941). Wait for me and I'll come back. *Pravda*, January 1942, A. Shlonsky (trans.).
Torok, M. (1986). Afterword: What is occult in occultism? Between Sigmund Freud and Sergei Pankeiev wolf man. In N. Abraham & M. Torok (Eds.) and N. Rand (Trans.), *The Wolf Man's magic word: A cryptonomy* (pp. 84–106). University of Minnesota Press.
Ullman, M. (2003). Dream telepathy: Experimental and clinical findings. In N. Totton (Ed.), *Psychoanalysis and the paranormal: Lands of darkness* (pp. 15–46). Karnac.
Winnicott, D. W. (1971). *Playing and reality.* Penguin.

Chapter 2

To Approach What Is Radically Other

Ofra Eshel's "Where Are You, My Beloved?"

Mary Tennes

Mary Tennes, Ph.D, an American psychoanalyst from the West Coast and a faculty member of the Psychoanalytic Institute of Northern California (PINC) comments on Ofra's chapter by highlighting how Ofra has fashioned throughout her psychoanalytic work an appeal for the analyst to be open to communication with the patient, and how Ofra's desire for openness has lent itself to the exploration of telepathy. In particular, Mary casts a wider net, prompted by the fact that her preparation for comments on Ofra's work occurred at the same time as the October 7, 2023 massacre in Israel. She wonders how we as a species communicate unconsciously with one another and contends that the existence of telepathy challenges us to "surrender to the loss of known ways of understanding and being."

* * * *

The morning of October 7, 2023, I sat down to begin writing this discussion of Ofra's paper, since the conference at which we were originally presenting was scheduled to be held a few months later. I opened my computer and wrote a first paragraph in which I was appreciating the chance to speak about her compelling presentation. Through her gifts as a clinician, writer, and scholar, I said, Ofra has played a central role in opening and substantiating the exploration of telepathic and other uncanny phenomena within psychoanalysis. She locates these experiences within a revolutionary approach to analytic work in which, extending Winnicott's and Bion's most radical ideas, she emphasizes the profound interconnectedness between patient and analyst (Eshel, 2019).

Suddenly, the news began to flash across my screen that Hamas had attacked Israel, and the horror and grief of what was happening began to unfold. Ofra was in Tel Aviv, her home. I wrote to her; she said that she had been in a bomb shelter but had just emerged. The trauma, grief, shock, and dismay of the situation was overwhelming. I stopped writing. And, in the days following, I continued to struggle with what to write. The atrocities of these unprecedented attacks left me wordless. In the wake of this disastrous situation, our conference was postponed.

Clearly, my discussion had suddenly been altered by the mind-boggling intersection of beginning to write at the moment Ofra was suddenly and literally under siege. Rather than having the luxury of focusing only on Ofra's

DOI: 10.4324/9781003611042-3

paper, I now had to address these colliding realities: an exploration of analytic moments of "oneness," as Ofra calls them, between patient and analyst side by side with the most horrific moments of disconnectedness and Othering between one people and another. How to hold together these seemingly impossible-to-integrate events? One might think that talking about telepathic dreams between patient and analyst is a cloistered conversation in the face of a world in which people are being recklessly annihilated. In contrast, I see these profound moments within analytic work as urgently relevant to the question of how we contend with the collective catastrophes we are now facing. I will attempt, by the end of this discussion, to make that link.

One place to begin is with the fact of being changed by experiences that unexpectedly present themselves to us. This discussion, over time, has required an ongoing adaptation to the circumstances that have arisen. As the disastrous situation in the Middle East and the responses to it became dramatically, tragically heightened, I felt the need to revise what I said several times. And now, again, given all that continues to unfold, both there and here in our country, I have continued to contemplate changes.

The fact of being altered is also at the heart of a conversation about telepathic and uncanny experiences within psychoanalysis. Awe-inspiring clinical moments like the telepathic dream that Ofra describes challenge our everyday convictions about sensory reality and disrupt the familiar ground upon which we orient and stand. They are shocking, frightening, amazing—and so inevitably invite the analyst and the analysis itself to open to the unknown. Such openness is not so easy.

In fact, the exploration of the telepathic has, throughout the history of psychoanalysis, been foreclosed with great force. Beginning with Freud, analysts who have experienced the startling, inexplicable quality of telepathic and other uncanny clinical moments have frequently hidden these experiences for fear of risking their professional reputations (Mayer & Stoller, 2001). Freud himself insisted that his early experiments with Ferenczi and Jung on "thought-transference" between patient and analyst be kept secret, for fear that their exposure would cause "the psychoanalytic house to explode" (Freud, 1925, p. 209). When analysts in the decades after Freud have attempted to report such occurrences, they have most frequently been viewed through a denigrating, rejecting lens: as unscientific, defensive, naive, regressed, or even mad (Eshel, 2006). In a field that purports to be scientific, the need to turn away from experiences that challenge the existing paradigm is a striking statement about the threats they pose.

Of course, it can be highly threatening to let go of the ground upon which we base our conceptualizations of ourselves and the world. Yet doing so is, in a sense, the premise and the power of a psychoanalytic approach: to work through our defenses against that which might unravel our known identifications. In particular, the unnerving reality that telepathic phenomena expose is one of incomprehensible interconnectedness, analogous to what physicists refer to as "quantum entanglement," a proven yet still unexplained phenomenon in which two particles mysteriously act as if they were one entity even if separated by great distances (Bass, 2001;

Dillow, 2016). To truly open oneself to a telepathic dream in which self and other are somehow mysteriously, inexplicably connected is to open oneself to experiences that upend our known, collective assumptions about reality and selfhood. And I believe that the courage to open to the recognition of astounding interconnectedness between human beings offers a pathway to begin to counteract the blind and terrifying dehumanization that we are now witnessing globally.

So how do we not turn away from that which poses a threat to our established ways of knowing? Ofra offers herself as an example of both the inevitable hesitation and the necessary courage involved. She tells us that in response to the first two telepathic dreams that patients brought to her, she "pushed them to some remote corner of [her] mind" (Eshel, 2024, p. 3), and only later, when three more such dreams entered into her practice, did she allow herself to face the incomprehension and discomfort they evoked. She quotes Pontalis (2003), who speaks of "allow[ing] ourselves to be touched, wounded, and demolished in our own being … in order to try to approach what is radically other" (Eshel, 2024, p. 4). In beginning with this focus, Ofra highlights the profound receptivity that such moments require. In order to be true to our analytic enterprise, we must allow ourselves to be affected, de-integrated, unraveled. Like a caterpillar who, entering into a transformative cocooning process, literally turns itself into liquid, we are challenged to surrender to the loss of known ways of understanding and being.

In taking up this challenge, Ofra describes the case of Effie, for whom the traumatic legacy of the Holocaust became a haunting presence. Part of what I find fascinating about Ofra's presentation of Effie's history are the words she both uses and doesn't use to describe the central events. Effie's mother and grandmother, she says, fled from Poland, but the mother's father and husband, along with the rest of the family, "were caught and sent to concentration camps, where they perished" (Eshel, 2024, p. 5). These last words are definitive, as though the deaths have been confirmed. And yet, a few paragraphs later, we hear that when Effie was ten months old, "her mother's first husband suddenly reappeared" (p. 6). In a way that must reproduce Effie's experience, there is no commentary or explanation about the discrepancy between the original certainty and the new reality that presents itself, so that the supposedly dead husband's sudden arrival shocks and confuses, leaving the listener in a kind of gap or limbo. Through this wording, the ex-husband seems to appear like a ghost out of nowhere.

On the one hand, Ofra's conscious or unconscious use of language mirrors and evokes the dissociative disjuncture of the traumatic, the breach that occurs in the face of the unbearable. Like an apparition caught in the gap between life and death, Effie herself feels "stuck somewhere in the middle" (Eshel, 2024, pp. 10–11). Ofra had to "hold her firmly, lest she slip away through the empty spaces in her words" (p. 11). Entering into a state of "at-one-ment" with Effie, Ofra doesn't simply describe her patient, but also recreates Effie's experience so that we as listeners feel it as well.

And yet I also think this interesting absence of explanatory language speaks to the topic Ofra has taken up: the difficulty contending with that which, like a telepathic dream, defies understanding. A telepathic dream arrives like an apparition: unsettling, spooky, enigmatic, disrupting the known framework of things. It challenges us to be receptive to that which unravels our understanding. And that is what Ofra does, listening "in astonishment" (Eshel, 2024, p. 13) to the dream details that mirror her own experience, not retreating from the inexplicable.

On a Wednesday—the day of the week that Ofra and Effie didn't meet—Effie dreamed of going at four o'clock to the cemetery where her father was buried. She saw a beautiful picture of him and experienced a new feeling of longing. That same Wednesday, Ofra went at four o'clock to the cemetery where her own father was being memorialized; she had been especially missing him at this time and felt intense longing. The telepathic link between Effie and Ofra and between dream and reality is stunning. What is also remarkable is that the other details of the dream play out between Ofra and her patient as they are being shared between them. Effie tells Ofra she had been feeling detached the previous two days when they met, and she thought that Ofra had been detached as well, something Ofra realizes is true. In the dream, Effie sees that the gate she must go through is closing, but she is able to persuade the gatekeeper to keep it open and let her in. Ofra, it seems, was a gate that was closing. In a beautifully skillful clinical exchange, she addresses Effie's ghostlike detachment—in response to her own detachment—encouraging her to "come back down to me and tell me what's happening" (Eshel, 2024, p. 11). Then, as Effie describes the dream, Ofra allows herself to be profoundly affected and altered by what she hears, becoming the gatekeeper who lets the gate open again. Effie is not only presenting a dream; she and Ofra are living the dream together as it is being told.

Part of what is so astounding about telepathic dreams is that they expose a mysterious, uncanny interconnectedness not only between patient and analyst, but also between states of dreaming and waking. When the dream world and the waking world seem to touch, our everyday orientation to reality is challenged. Our assumptions about the separateness of self and other and of internal and external worlds, as well as our established sense of time and space, are momentarily suspended.

Current scientific discoveries support such paradigm-altering revisions in our orientation. In a beautiful article exploring the parallels between the theories of Wilfred Bion and those of physicist David Bohm, Robert Godwin (1991) notes that one of the "bewildering abstrusities" of contemporary physics is that its equations describe realities "which literally [cannot] be pictured in the mind; for the first time in history, science [has] produced a model of the universe which [is] beyond our ability to comprehend" (p. 627). Bohm himself suggests that in order to approach an accurate understanding of reality, our familiar ways of conceptualizing have to be suspended. Our normal categories of thought, he says, cannot do justice to that which we are attempting to grasp. In his words, "the dissolution of thinking … is the highest priority the seeker for truth can undertake" to be replaced by what he calls “intelligence” (quoted in Godwin p. 634). This movement is akin to Bion’s idea that the analyst must, each session, suspend memory and desire in order to release saturated forms of thinking and to be present for the new patient arriving each hour. In fact, Tom Ogden (2015) suggests that if we actually grasp what Bion is asking of us, we should be “stunned” (p. 291).

And indeed, Bohm proposes a stunning, mind-altering model of the universe that requires a relinquishment of our most fundamental assumptions. The perceived world of separate, fragmented entities, he says, is merely a surface manifestation of an underlying “fundamental realm of unbroken wholeness” (Godwin, 1991, p. 628) out of which the sensory world of individual identities emerges. The world of difference, as we perceive it, Bohm says, is more holographic than fixed and substantial; interconnectedness is the foundational reality.

Contemporary science, in fact, has leapt remarkably past its Newtonian origins so that, as Sean Carroll, a prominent physicist, says:

> Quantum mechanics … is one of the most impressive intellectual accomplishments in the entire history of the human race … because every idea … violate (s) some cherished notion that we had really clung to. We had this paradigm handed down by Galileo and Newton and that was how physics was done … and quantum mechanics comes along and changes all of the rules.
>
> (S. Carroll, personal communication, 2024)

Psychoanalysis is similarly challenged to let go of the Newtonian origins that framed Freud’s model of the mind. Telepathic dreams disrupt us not only in a momentary and personal way within the analytic encounter; they also challenge certain cherished psychoanalytic convictions.

From that vantage point, I would like to take up a complexity in Ofra’s paper. On the one hand, she emphasizes the inexplicable mystery she encountered in hearing her patients’ telepathic dreams, and she herself makes links to mind-boggling scientific discoveries, referring to Bohm and to the “quantum interconnectedness” such dreams expose, “defying space, time, and personal boundaries” (Eshel, 2024, p. 23). But then, in an interesting turn, she attempts to “unravel and understand these enigmatic, abstruse phenomena” (p. 16) by explaining their occurrence as an expression of an archaic mode of communication in patients whose parents were traumatically absent. In defending against a return to such devastating loss, she says, the patient creates a telepathic dream, a pre-verbal mode of functioning that, like a search engine, reaches out to find the analyst.

Although I would be hesitant to assume that all telepathic dreams arise in the context of traumatic early experience, I too had a patient with a history of unbearable maternal absence who brought an astounding telepathic dream to me, and, when I let her know about the shocking links between her dream and my life, she burst into tears, saying “we are so connected!” (Tennes, 2024). These uncanny moments clearly can function within the treatment to reveal a deep and startling bond between patient and analyst when a profound connection may feel urgently necessary. I also think these dreams can often function, as they did with Ofra's patient, to disrupt and move the analyst into new forms of awareness and relatedness. Furthermore, the link between the shattering effects of trauma and the receptivity to experiences that dislodge the cohesiveness of our everyday orientation to reality is a territory that could use further exploration.

At the same time, I would make a distinction between exploring the function of telepathic dreams within any analysis and attempting to explain the awe-inspiring, disruptive realities they present. The reason such experiences have been so sequestered for decades is because they disrupt the familiar ground of our psychoanalytic paradigm and ask us to bear the absence of a framework within which to encompass them. A familiar concept like "unconscious communication" does not explain how such phenomena occur, any more than the terms "quantum entanglement" or "spooky action at a distance" explain the unanswered mystery of intertwined particles. Furthermore, equating uncanny, telepathic experiences with primitive forms of psychological functioning can move away from something more startling about them. In archaic, pre-verbal modes of communication, self and other lose their separateness as a certain merger or fusion is sought. Telepathic moments, however, are often characterized by a quality of paradox in which self and other both are and are not separate. When my patient, stunned, said "we are so connected," she was awestruck by the fact that while being two distinct subjects, like two particles at a distance, we were nonetheless, somehow, in a profound, inexplicable alignment.

When a telepathic dream arises in a treatment, we are challenged to remain open to its disorienting effects. Ofra, in fact, has an exceptional gift for this kind of clinical presence. Her book, *The Emergence of Analytic Oneness* (Eshel, 2019), provides numerous examples of her capacity to risk familiar, comfortable analytic positioning in order to enter into the primal disturbance her patients bring to her and, in so doing, to transform what could otherwise seem to be intractable difficulties. Ironically, psychoanalytic theory itself is being similarly challenged to move out of familiar ground in order to be transformed by the mysteries that telepathic moments present.

To return to the beginning of my discussion, I see this capacity to let go of the known and to open to what is "radically other" as profoundly relevant to the seemingly intractable disturbances of our world. Our temptation, in the face of that which threatens us, is to retreat to established ways of seeing and, in solidifying our own identities, to view the other as Other. Any awareness of interconnectedness is lost as we entrench our egoic patterns and move more readily into states of certainty, anger, control, and domination. So how do we counteract these all-too-human tendencies? How can we bring a psychoanalytic sensibility to bear on the terrible destructiveness we are currently witnessing?

At the beginning of her book, in describing the analyst's capacity to enter into an analytic process, Ofra, using a biblical phrase from King Solomon, refers to the "the hearing heart" (Eshel, 2019, p. 11). As psychoanalysts, she says, we move into states of oneness with our patients by daring to open our hearts to "the heart-break which is at the centre of human existence" (p. 13). Psychoanalytic listening, she suggests, comes from a heart willing to be altered, even shattered, by what it hears. Ofra herself demonstrates this willingness in a way that provides a profound and compelling model for clinical work. And our own courage to bring such open-heartedness not only to our patients, but also to the devastating global realities we are contending with, is a path of transformation offered by psychoanalysis at its best.

In fact, I see telepathic dreams less as extraordinary phenomena than as momentary windows that open, allowing us to see what we ordinarily do not see: a deep, abiding interconnectedness between us underlying the divisions we so readily perceive and create. The path of openness is not an easy one; but it does, in our work and in our world, seem essential.

References

Bass, A. (2001). It takes one to know one; Or, whose unconscious is it anyway? *Psychoanalytic Dialogues*, 11, 683–702.

Dillow, C. (2016, March 30). *Quantum entanglement: Action at a distance.* Retrieved from www.space.com/31933-quantum-entanglement-action-at-a-distance.html.

Eshel, O. (2006). Where are you, my beloved? *International Journal of Psychoanalysis*, 87, 1603–1627.

Eshel, O. (2019). *The emergence of analytic oneness: Into the heart of psychoanalysis.* Routledge.

Eshel, O. (2024). Where are you, my beloved: On absence, loss, and the enigma of telepathic dreams. Presented at IPTAR Conference on Telepathy, June 2024.

Freud, S. (1925). Letter from Sigmund Freud to Sándor Ferenczi, March 20, 1925. In E. Falzeder & E. Brabant (Eds.), *The correspondence of Sigmund Freud and Sándor Ferenczi, 1920–1933* (Vol. 3, pp. 209–210). Harvard University Press.

Godwin, R. W. (1991). Wilfred Bion and David Bohm: Toward a quantum metapsychology. *Psychoanalysis and Contemporary Thought*, 14, 625–654.

Mayer, E. L., & Stoller, R. J. (2001). On "Telepathic dreams?" An unpublished paper by Robert J. Stoller. *Journal of the American Psychoanalytic Association*, 49, 629–657.

Ogden, T. H. (2015). Intuiting the truth of what's happening: On Bion's "Notes on memory and desire." *Psychoanalytic Quarterly*, 84, 285–306.

Pontalis, J. B. (2003). *Windows* (A. Quinney, Trans.). University of Nebraska Press.

Tennes, M. (2024). Tell all the truth but tell it slant: Psychoanalysis and the uncanny. *Contemporary Psychoanalysis*, 60, 146–166.

Chapter 3

Piercing the Veil

From Intuition to Telepathic Receptivity

Janine de Peyer

Janine de Peyer, LCSW., a relational psychoanalyst from the National Institute for the Psychotherapies (NIP) in New York City provides one of the most poignant examples of dream telepathy of a patient who picks up on an immediate frightening medical event of Janine's husband the previous night, except that the patient dreams the event occurred to her own husband. In addition, another of Janine's patients appeared to telepathically communicate to Janine the name of a mother figure who had been important in her early development. Despite the fact that in this last instance, the patient fit the description of someone who grew up with a distant and inattentive mother, Janine contends that this paradigm does not always take place and cites yet another experience of hers. She concludes; "a feeling of intense emotional absence or loss is not always a necessary precursor for a telepathic transmission."

* * * *

How do we really speak to one another, and how do we listen? In clinical work, who's doing the speaking, and who is doing the listening? In contemporary psychoanalysis, the illusory boundary between self and other is being increasingly challenged. What's yours, what's mine, and do we even know the difference? When confronted with an apparent telepathic transmission, the experience of separation between self and other evaporates, forcing both analyst and patient into mutual surrender to an alternate reality of psychic interconnectivity.

Acceptance of the existence of telepathic interconnectivity means, by implication, accepting that we live in a potentially boundaryless world unlimited by space and time. This level of psychic interconnectivity sometimes represents a "portal" offering new possibilities of clinical transformation (de Peyer, 2021). Such porousness can also, however, feel unsettling and weirdly destabilizing for both clinician and patient (de Peyer, 2022).

I will present examples from two clinical cases, illustrating how unbidden telepathic, clairvoyant, or precognitive information can penetrate our analytic space, eliciting differing reactions in the same analyst. I place these different telepathic communications on a "continuum of mutual receptivity and human

DOI: 10.4324/9781003611042-4

empathic responsiveness" (de Peyer, 2014, p. 112). This continuum attempts to delineate varying levels of telepathic receptivity. On one end of this continuum, I place non-telepathic, explicitly verbal, seemingly conscious levels of oral and physical communications. An example would be offering a verbally empathic response when it is obvious that the patient is upset. Moving along the continuum, we might place sensory based, less conscious, more intuitive communications, such as picking up somatic cues that the patient is upset, even when the patient's affect appears blunted or numb. Next, we might place nonverbal, unconscious, projective exchanges such as projective identifications (de Peyer, 2017), where the analyst might unwittingly pick up and embody evacuated feelings/thoughts that are dissociated and projected by the patient within a session. Finally, on the far end of this continuum, I would place nonlocal, paranormal events, such as telepathic dreams or uncanny precognitions—where the analyst or patient knows something in detail about the other that has occurred between sessions, before, during, or after it has happened—without any logical way of knowing or access to sensory involvement.

As clinicians, we vary in our openness to belief in telepathy, fluctuating between acceptance and skepticism depending on our state of mind, our need for concrete evidence, or perhaps our sense of vulnerability vis-à-vis the unknown. For some, the idea that one can have a predictive dream, or telepathically "know" another person's thoughts without any sensory communication, feels like a stretch. The long history of criticism of telepathy research (Wiseman & Watt, 2004) largely focuses on its lack of controls, or due to the unpredictability of telepathic exchange, results are not found to be replicated in subsequent studies. Within psychoanalysis, reports of telepathic transmissions are unavoidably subjective personal accounts, making them impossible to prove and therefore open to being debunked. Nonetheless, reports within psychoanalysis are multiplying (Rabeyron et al., 2020), and interest is growing. I suggest that, given the intensity of the therapeutic matrix, we open our minds, pay serious attention to this proliferation of reports, and consider that psychic interconnectedness may indeed underlie all therapeutic endeavors, existing as a constant, exerting its timeless influence outside our conscious awareness, until an unbidden telepathic exchange pierces our veil of consensus "reality." We might have varying degrees of receptivity to having this veil pierced, but, as the saying goes, adapted from William James (1909),[1] "We are like islands in the sea, separate on the surface but connected in the deep."

Prior to experiencing unbidden anomalous exchanges in my clinical work, a handful of unexplainable, uncanny events had taken place in my personal life over the course of three decades. These events undoubtedly stimulated my curiosity about the nature of implicit human interconnectedness, but I had nonetheless remained dubious and wary of "cult-like" beliefs in the supernatural. One such early example that caught my attention, however, was in my early twenties, when sitting in a laundromat watching my washing going round and around, I simply "knew" that the young man whom I loved, and with whom six weeks earlier I'd had a rupture resulting in break-up, was at that very moment on his way to my house. I dropped what I was doing, left my clothes circling in the machine, and raced home to arrive at my front gate at the precise moment when my ex-boyfriend arrived on foot from the opposite direction. How had I "known" he was on his way to my house? How do we explain experiences such as these?

I will share one more unexplainable personal event before turning to clinical illustrations. One morning I awoke in my New York City apartment having had a dream about a woman I had met at college in England ten years earlier. I had not been particularly close to this woman, and I'd had no contact with her for ten years. "Why on earth am I dreaming about Sally?" I wondered. I left my apartment, walked to the subway station, went down the steps to the express platform, and who was standing right there next to me—Sally—on a tourist visit to New York. The fact that I had just dreamt about her without having seen or spoken to her in ten years, and that I'd *remembered* my dream minutes before actually running into her, astounded me. Is it possible that my psyche somehow energetically picked up Sally's physical presence in New York City, and with an uncanny prescience, anticipated running into her in my dream?

For many years, I kept events like these to myself fearing dismissal or judgment, but when a series of telepathic transmissions began occurring with a patient of mine I call "Jordan," my intellectual curiosity caught fire, compelling me to dive headlong into telepathy research. This research resulted in the publication, "Uncanny Communication and the Porous Mind" (de Peyer, 2016a). I will summarize here some of the anomalous events that took place between Jordan and me in order to contrast these anomalous occurrences with a second clinical case, which similarly involved the uncanny choice of a name. I will examine and contrast these two cases, placing them along a continuum of telepathic mutual receptivity, while also delving into the transference–countertransference conundrums the clinician faces when confronted by such unbidden telepathic exchanges.

I felt compelled to publish on this controversial topic because the hypothesized existence of the paranormal challenges implicit assumptions that have been carried down through generations of orthodoxy in the sciences and in psychology. Those interested in parapsychology, dating back to William James (1902) and J. B. Rhine (1934), have followed their curiosity into uncharted territory with conviction, despite facing vehement criticism every step of the way. As the topic of telepathic interconnectedness is now gaining traction both in psychoanalytic literature and conference presentations (e.g., The William Alanson White Institute, NY, Colloquium Series, 2021–22; and IPTAR's May 2024 two-day conference, "A Century of Mystery: Telepathy in the Clinical Process"), I have grown emboldened to write about both personal and clinical uncanny communications, realizing that the "porousness" exhibited by such experiences offers a heightened sensibility that, when developed, can serve as a useful intuitive guide in clinical work.

Sadly, Freud's (1901, 1933) retreat from his initial interest in telepathy and thought transference, due to his need to protect psychoanalysis from association with superstition, religiosity, or the paranormal (Massicotte, 2014), meant that psychoanalysis largely went dark on this subject for many decades. His famous recommendation to avoid such "dangerous expeditions" (Brabant et al., 1992, p. 274) carries enduring influence to this day. I believe Freud's ensuing reluctance to publicly pursue his interest in telepathy left an indelible stain on the psychoanalytic imagination. Here we are, more than one hundred years later, still skeptical about considering the existence of anomalous, "psychic" forms of communication (Cardeña et al., 2014), many in our field still preferring to use euphemistic, blanket statement terms such as "unconscious communication," or "unconscious to unconscious," rather than more direct, explicit terms such as "telepathic," "anomalous," or "paranormal" to distinguish nonlocal telepathic transmissions from sensory-based forms of intuitive communication. Patients who report telepathic experiences to mental health professionals are still routinely assessed for psychosis (Beyer, 2017; Greyson, 1977), and decades of valuable research collaboration between parapsychologists and psychologists have been delayed or, worse, systematically dismissed (Alcock, 1998; Luckhurst, 2023; Wiseman, 1997; Wiseman & Watt, 2004).

The area of parapsychology research that has nevertheless most readily captured our twenty-first-century psychoanalytic imagination centers on telepathic dreams between patients and their analysts (Eshel, 2006; Mayer, 2001; Suchet, 2004; Ullman, 2003). Here, it is sleep that facilitates the emergence of transcendental material: it is our dreamworld that beckons us across the threshold into the paranormal. Telepathic communications occurring during *wakefulness*, however, especially between people who are geographically separated from one another, continue to pose a greater challenge within psychoanalysis, since they require a stark deviation from mainstream, Western, Newtonian-based, beliefs about "reality."

What Creates Psychic At-tune-ment?

Many theorists (such as Frankel, 2004) believe that developmental trauma, or environmental disruption, creates a hyper-vigilance that can contribute to humans' increased intuitive porousness. Although this often appears to be the case in clinical work, I support additional researchers' views (such as Carson et al., 2003), who suspect that being raised in an atmosphere of nonverbal creativity (such as musicians/visual artists/filmmakers/dancers) might also heighten one's receptivity to anomalous forms of communication, enhancing one's capacity for "tuning-in." Growing up in a family of musicians in a British household where music, rather than the spoken language, was the primary mode of emotional expression primed me, I believe, to "listen" empathically, tuning in beyond words. Children also seem to have a particular radar for anomalous forms of communication, and perhaps the loosening of cognition so innate to playfulness and creative expression enhances one's capacity for telepathic receptivity. In adults, the minimization of sensory distractions, engagement in meditation practices, focused visualization, or the pursuit of transcendent states (Mascaro et al., 2013; Radin, 2013), along with the heightening of one's empathic connections and belief in the possibility of "psi," all potentially increase the likelihood that telepathic exchange might penetrate through to conscious awareness.

The Case of "Jordan"

The series of synchronistic exchanges between Jordan and me began with the uncanny transmission of a name (de Peyer, 2016a, 2016b, 2022). Jordan, an anxious, White, cisgender, heterosexual woman in her late thirties, had been planning for a long time to leave New York to attend a week-long photography retreat in Santa Fe, New Mexico. I had been treating her for about 18 months, focusing mainly on self-regulation and management of turbulent transference-countertransference dynamics leading to frequent ruptures and repairs. Married, and recently having helped her husband through a serious illness, Jordan was now eager to reconnect with her own passion for photography. Her husband, now fully recovered, was encouraging her to go.

Jordan had grown up in a family with dysregulated rage and physical violence—her father would beat her older brother, who would then routinely beat Jordan. She lived in a constant state of hyper-vigilance, afraid to come home from school to be alone in the house with her brother who would terrorize, spit, hit, and kick her before her parents would get home. She would later be blamed by her parents for somehow having provoked her brother, leaving Jordan feeling dejected, unprotected, and alone. This environment led her to develop a tough veneer, protecting a vulnerable core self that could easily become destabilized. In our work together, Jordan vehemently disdained any hint of dependency on me. She was highly critical, prone to affective storms, and demanding of my closest attentiveness. Our transference-countertransference dynamic would take center stage most sessions, leaving little time for fact-gathering, or attention to concrete details about her life, such as names, dates, or places. As I learned to better attune to her fears and we worked through repeated ruptures and repairs, she was increasingly able to regulate her anger, and her marriage began to stabilize.

As the date of her photography retreat in Santa Fe approached, she was getting cold feet. We'd been discussing her desire for this trip for many months. The trip had great symbolic meaning for Jordan, signaling a return to independence after her husband's recovery, and a reclaiming of her own talents and creative aspirations. She had worked through many of her fears about leaving, but one June morning—right before the trip—she was once more hesitating. She was seized with doubt. Without realizing it, I had found myself caught in a transference-countertransference enactment in which I'd become overly invested in Jordan's bid for independence and creative exploration, temporarily losing my empathic connection with her fearful, more vulnerable child part. Perhaps exhausted at this point from her repeated ruminations and reversals, I'd been feeling a growing sense of exasperation and disappointment. Her associations in the session drifted to her childhood fears, reliving, yet again, frightening scenes with her brother in which she would struggle to protect herself. This time, however, she shared with me that as a child she'd finally found a solution to her problem: she started going home every day from school to her best friend Alicia's house in the next town, a sanctuary where she could wait until her parents would pick her up on their way home. She could thus avoid being alone in the house with her brother and avoid her parents' blame and recrimination when they finally got home.

After recounting this childhood memory, Jordan's associations jumped back to the photographic retreat, and she dug her heels in:

> "I just can't go! I can't get on that plane … Santa Fe is just too far away!" she said.
>
> "It's not about the geography!" I exclaimed, feeling a surge of frustration. "You could always text or Facetime with him from there … You could be in … Tuckahoe for that matter, and still talk it through with him!"
>
> "Tuckahoe?" Where had that name come from, I wondered? I had been trying to say "Timbuktu!" Jordan then had a quizzical look on her face.
>
> "How did you know that's the name of the town where my friend Alicia lived?" she said, "… the town I've been talking about here for the past half hour?"

We both realized I had somehow come up with the very name of the place where she'd go to feel safe after school, without her ever having mentioned it. I had never actually heard of the town "Tuckahoe" and had no idea how that name had popped out of my mouth. A strange feeling came over my body—an invisible boundary had just been crossed between us. I saw the hint of a smile flit across Jordan's face. I asked what she made of me coming up with that name?

> "Oh, that sort of thing happens to me all the time," she said, "People just know things … and I just know things about people."

The sudden intrusion of this name shocked us out of our impasse and had a detoxifying, containing effect on both of us. It wasn't until later that I realized the image of Tuckahoe symbolically represented the heart of her current dilemma: how to take care of herself—leaving home in a way that could feel safe, while also retaining her primary attachments (in this case, to her husband and to me). Through the sudden intrusion of the name "Tuckahoe," it was as if our two psyches had become linked at a critical moment of impasse, offering a "paranormal solution" (Rabeyron et al., 2021) that called us back together. This "solution" provided an elegant and cogent interpretation more precise than anything I could have conjured up consciously, especially while in a state of heightened countertransference activation. Some form of psychic "melding" had provided us with the answer. I didn't know at that moment that this would be the first of several uncanny exchanges between us.

After my initial reaction of astonishment, privately I felt myself recoil slightly with uneasiness. My relationship with Jordan had not been easy. Despite my own prior personal experiences with the uncanny and a general open-mindedness to the concept of telepathy, I nonetheless felt uncomfortable experiencing this degree of porousness with a patient. I was fascinated by what had happened, yet it felt as if the boundaries of the psychoanalytic frame that I'd worked so hard to maintain with her were evaporating. Did I really want this degree of unconscious fusion with Jordan's inner world?

Searching for Telepathic Allies

After many years of reflection, I can now see how fragile I was in those early days of writing about this case. There were only a few psychoanalytic clinicians who had had the courage to publish on anomalous transmission (e.g., Altman, 2002; Bass, 2001; Eshel, 2006; Rosenbaum, 2011; Schwarz, 1969; Suchet, 2004; Tennes, 2007). As I searched for allies, I was encouraged by Freud's (1923) initial interest in telepathy and his conviction that through the analyst's "evenly suspended attention," one can "catch the drift" of the patient's unconscious with one's own unconscious (p. 239). I became fascinated by the question of *just how much* both patient and analyst are able to pick up on one another's unconscious. What drifts or fantasies, physical sensations, or mental distractions of our own are patients able to perceive, and what does this mean about the privacy (or lack thereof) of our countertransference? I found comfort in Ferenczi's (1988) notion of the "dialogue of unconsciouses" (p. 84) that captured something of the uncanny flow between Jordan and me—a flow that Bollas (1995) poetically describes as the "discordant symphonic movement" of a "reciprocally infinite falling of one self, into another" (p. 28).

By contrast, Freud's (1912) analogy of the telephone receiver[2] upheld a *directional* theory of unconscious communication where one person "sends" something to another. Projective identification was also initially depicted as uni-directional, where the patient "sent" evacuated feelings to the analyst to metabolize (Bion, 1962). A bi-directional notion of *mutual* unconscious reciprocity, on the other hand, challenges traditionally held notions of analytic hierarchy, dissolving the illusory boundary between self and other and calling into question the analyst's capacity to choose between consciously intended versus unintentional self-disclosures. Findings from recent neuroscientific research and neuroimaging technology—such as Berlin (2011), Gallese (2006, 2009), McGilchrist (2009), and Schore (2003)—also suggest that our brains are mutually capable of reading other brains in subtle, complex ways, far beyond our conscious comprehension. So how do we understand the means by which one human brain unconsciously transmits precise information such as a name across a room to another human brain? And how far does right-hemisphere to right-hemisphere communication travel, anyway? Might this unconscious "reading" somehow take place constantly, mutually and simultaneously at all times, beyond our conscious awareness and even beyond geographical proximity?

Since Freud's introduction of the telephone analogy, less directional metaphors that capture the mutual co-resonance demonstrated by telepathic communication are represented by Winnicott's (1975) "transitional space," Searles' (1973) "symbiotic relatedness," Ogden's (1997) "intersubjective analytic third," Baranger and Baranger's (2008) "dynamic field," and Civitarese and Ferro's (2013) "bi-personal field." These metaphors all attempt to capture the reciprocity and permeability involved with telepathic interconnectedness. Elizabeth Lloyd Mayer's *Extraordinary Knowing* (2007) offers a widely comprehensive survey of research into this scientifically "inexplicable" psychic porousness. By linking Freud's original ideas on telepathy with reports on CIA experiments on remote viewing, cutting-edge neuroscientific experimentation, and evolving theories from quantum physics, Mayer forwards convincing arguments in favor of the acceptance of the existence of "psi" phenomena. To my mind, however, it is Bion's (1970) concept of "transformation in O" that most accurately describes the overwhelming clinical experience of utter surrender to uncertainty that one feels when struck by an uncanny transmission—a total emotional immersion, or "being-in-oneness," at a primordial point of origin (Eshel, 2016).

With the introduction of Heisenberg's (1927) uncertainty principle (the impossibility of measuring position, speed, and trajectory of a particle simultaneously), along with the "observer effect" (the notion that the act of observing influences the observed), uni-directional metaphors within psychoanalysis have conceded to notions of bi-directionality, which are now more widely accepted in two-person, intersubjective models of psychoanalysis (Aron, 1990). Therefore, rather than holding the view that Jordan somehow "sent" me or "planted" the name "Tuckahoe" in my mind, I prefer the view that I "borrowed a thought" or tapped into shared archetypal imagery of a sanctuary in the form of "Tuckahoe" from a unified field of knowledge; a shared consciousness—or as Carl Jung (1959) might put it, from the collective unconscious.

Perhaps it is time to consider a "three-person psychology" or a "psychoanalytic third" that includes the uncanny. If we apply the quantum mechanics metaphor of interaction between two particles to the interaction between minds, two or more minds might then be viewed as "entangled" in an interconnectivity that transcends space and time. If Dean Radin (2006), the parapsychologist, is correct and human minds are indeed "entangled," this too suggests that a resonant interconnectedness might be available to us all at all times to process emotions in a shared, alternative realm of consciousness.

The Clinician's Responsiveness to Telepathic Involvement

My response to this first telepathic exchange between Jordan and me hovered between captivation and dread. When it is the patient who reports/introduces a telepathic word or dream, the clinician typically reacts in one of three ways:

1 Open-mindedness, supporting with curiosity the patient's expanded view of reality.
2 Incredulity, with an effort nonetheless to support the patient's subjective experience.
3 Discomfort and judgment, with uncertainty about how to handle it, possibly defensively judging or pathologizing the patient for their beliefs.

Reactions vary widely, of course, depending on one's predisposition to belief/disbelief in the paranormal and relationship with the particular patient involved. However, when it is the therapist him- or herself who has produced the breakthrough telepathic image, dream, or prescience (as with "Tuckahoe"), the shock can be particularly startling, since there is a feeling of loss of personal control—as if a "not me" self state has taken over (Bromberg, 2003) or one's own mind has been hijacked.

Further Anomalous Occurrences with "Jordan"

The Journey

Jordan had lent me a spiritual book called *The Journey* (Bays, 2014) that had been very meaningful to her, but which I had not yet found the time to read. I felt guilty about my delay in reading it and asked her at the end of a session one day if I could hold on to the book a while longer. "Sure," she said casually, saying I could keep it as long as I wanted. What she didn't tell me until many months later was that after she had left my office that day, the exact same book (which was not a bestseller or widely distributed) had "presented itself" to her twice within a couple of hours after leaving our session—first, in the cab ride going home when her husband brought up the book title out of the blue, and second, when riding the elevator up to her apartment she saw the same book tucked under her neighbor's arm. How are we to understand these reappearances? Coincidence? Synchronicity? Might my negligence at not having read the book have hurt her feelings, setting up some kind of resonant interconnectedness with her husband or even an acausal connectivity or psychokinetic convergence between mind and the material world involving her neighbor and his own copy of the book? A Western, Newtonian-based, material model of mind would balk at this latter suggestion.

Asking Permission

Once a number of these "coincidences" had occurred between Jordan and me, I started writing an academic paper about our uncanny interconnectivity, and I wanted to ask Jordan's permission to publish it. When finally having assessed that she'd be in a stable enough place to handle this disclosure, and believing that she might even be pleased by the idea, I was all set to ask her when she called requesting an emergency session. She anxiously wanted to discuss an "ethical dilemma" that she was facing about whether to publish a book of her own in which she needed to first ask "permission" from her own former clients to include photographs of interiors of their homes. I had no idea that she had been working on a book, and I had thus far disclosed nothing to her about writing my own paper. The synchronicity of her call felt uncannily competitive, as if she somehow wanted to pre-empt my publication with her own. I of course tabled my own request until she had comfortably resolved her own issue, only to share with her much later that we'd been entertaining the identical dilemma about "permission-seeking" at the very same time.

"Jordan's" Culminating Telepathic Dream

Up until this point, although somewhat eerie, our uncanny experiences had mostly felt exciting and intriguing to me. One Monday morning, however, my receptivity toward uncanny exchanges with Jordan took a turn. Jordan arrived early that morning, eager to recount a disturbing dream she had had during the weekend. In the dream, she had been fast asleep when she awakened to the sound of groans coming from her bathroom. Getting herself out of bed and running to the bathroom, she found her husband sitting on the toilet, head lowered in his hands, losing blood into the toilet bowl. She remembered waking up the following morning unsure if this had really happened or if it had just been a nightmare. She'd poked her husband and woke him up, asking him if he was alright or if it had just been a bad dream. He was fine. He put his arm around her and reassured her that thankfully rectal bleeding had never been one of the symptoms of his illness. They lay in bed together laughing, reveling in their shared relief.

What Jordan did not know (at least consciously) was that during that same night, the sound of disturbing groans had awakened *me* from my deep sleep, coming from my own bathroom. I had climbed out of bed and run to the bathroom where I'd found my own husband doubled over, head bowed, losing blood in the toilet bowl in the precise manner that Jordan had depicted. He was having an unprecedented medical emergency, exactly as Jordan had "seen" in her dream. Thankfully my husband's condition was later resolved, but that day, as Jordan recounted the dream to me, I could barely breathe, gripping the armrests on my chair in an attempt to ground myself.

This dream pushed the experience of boundarylessness between us to a new register. I did not tell her until much later what her dream had meant to me, but I wondered, how had I silently emitted this entire frightening scene to her during the night with such vivid detail? It felt like she had trespassed inside my mind—as if the privacy of my own bedroom had no boundary against her psychic invasions. Had she somehow unconsciously picked up on my fear that night during this episode? Was this telepathic dream stirred by concern and worry about me? Or did she feel abandoned by me—even angry—sensing my preoccupation and unavailability? This telepathic dream clearly defied all known boundaries of time and geographical space and shocked me to my core.

When examined as a group, the cumulative effect of these shared experiences between Jordan and me severely contested the possibility of "coincidence," coalescing into a repetitive pattern of uncanny transmission for which there was no material explanation. Each occurrence triggered different responses in me, ranging from intrigue and receptiveness to aversion and self-protective withdrawal. What was being communicated here? Did each telepathic exchange represent a specific transferential need? Was each anomalous transmission (through dyadic, psychic reenactment) pulling for the reenactment of a developmental wish, longing, or trauma belonging to either the patient, or myself? My varied response to each telepathic event raises the question: What function do telepathic transmissions play in clinical work?

The Case of "Diana"

I will now summarize a different case in which, again, the anomalous emergence of a name brought me closer to the patient, but this time proved pivotal to unlocking not only a moment of clinical impasse, but what had become a somewhat stymied treatment. Diana came to see me in the midst of an emotional crisis. A White, lesbian, cisgendered woman in her mid-forties, she'd been unhappily married to her wife for ten years with two small children. She had fallen in love with a female work associate with whom she'd been having an affair for two years. She came to treatment when her lover began to withdraw her interest, neglecting Diana, canceling their rendezvous, and behaving with increasing dismissiveness. Having previously felt enthralled by the relationship, Diana was now feeling anxious and bereft. Nervous about the potential of exiting her marriage, she'd wanted to protect the first name of her lover when we began our work together, so she'd asked me to come up with a name that we could call her lover. "Okay," I said, "Why don't we call her … I dunno … Florence?"

As we discussed her affair (referring to her lover as "Florence"), Florence was continuing to withdraw her attention, and Diana was becoming progressively devastated as she realized her two-year-long relationship with Florence was coming to an end. For the first time in her life, Diana had felt deeply known and understood by Florence—an experience she'd never felt with her wife. I began trying to explore Diana's childhood, searching for relational/attachment clues as to why she had picked a life partner with whom she'd never felt connected, and who she found vacuous and superficial when she longed for a deeper emotional engagement. In contrast, her secret relationship with Florence had felt so magical and deeply connected at the beginning, yet she was now finding herself constantly in the pursuer role, and Florence increasingly unavailable, and distracted.

Attempts I made to inquire into Diana's childhood came up dry. She had very few memories before adolescence. In fact, her entire childhood was presented as a blank. She reported that her parents had married when they were both twenty-one, and although they'd divorced when Diana was a teenager, she felt she'd had a decent enough childhood. It was hard to find developmental clues as to why Diana struggled so much in her own relational life. Diana remembered her mother as a physically beautiful woman, narcissistically self-involved, but nonetheless basically present most of the time and adequately administering to her needs. She also remembered that her mother was frequently on the phone (similar to her wife), but it was difficult to access negative feelings about her mother, beyond a hint of disdain. Although remaining close enough to her father, Diana's focus had always been on her peer relationships. She'd come out as queer in high school, had friends she could relate to, and she'd left for college as soon as she was old enough. She reported that neither parent seemed to have a problem with her sexuality, each having gay and lesbian friends within their own work/friendship circles. I could not get a textured sense of her childhood, and once in adulthood, Diana did not find it strange that she rarely saw her mother. She felt proud of the fact that she'd been super independent from early on in her life and moved to New York. The only emotional traction I could access in sessions centered on her emotional distress caused by her lover "Florence's" withdrawal.

One day, Diana arrived for her session telling me that her mother's lifelong best friend had reached out to her, concerned about her mother's drinking. This friend of her mother's had frequently been around when Diana was growing up, spending a lot of time in Diana's home. She met her mother's friend for coffee, and they talked. Because of our work together, Diana decided to ask the friend if she thought her mother had been a good mother to her. The friend proceeded to tell Diana a story.

One morning, when Diana was about two and a half years old, the friend came over to the house at around 11:30 am to have coffee with Diana's mother. There was no answer at the door. She banged loudly, then walked around the house and could see Diana's mother through the window, laying flat out on her bed, fast asleep. She banged repeatedly on the windowpane, calling out the mother's name, until finally her mother woke up and came to the front door. The friend then went to Diana's room where she found her lying alone in her crib, a half-empty bottle beside her, covered in urine and feces.

> "Florence told me," Diana continued, "that she picked me up from my crib and said, 'C'mere sweetie … I see you've peed and pooped all over…' to which Florence said I replied, 'I'm not s'posed to wake up mommy …'"

"Wait a minute ..." I said, "... Florence? Did you say Florence said she'd picked you up? Your mom's best friend's name is Florence?"

"Yea."

"... Like our Florence?" I said, taken aback. "You mean she had the same name as your lover?"

"Yes."

"Why didn't you ever tell me that?" I said. "Isn't that weird, for you, that all this time we've been using the same name for your lover as your mother's best friend?"

"Well I didn't pick that name," she said. "You did."

"I did?" I said, momentarily not remembering and doubting myself.

"Well I certainly wouldn't have picked the name Florence, would I?" she said.

"No. I guess not," I said, "but why didn't you say something when I picked that name?"

"I dunno," she said, "You picked 'Florence,' and I always liked my mother's best friend, so ... I guess I just went along with it."

I was thrown off for a moment, wondering why on earth I would have picked an old-fashioned name like "Florence" anyway for this young woman's lover, but vaguely remembering spontaneously coming up with it. Still, I had no prior association to this name. Diana then went on to recount that her mother's friend, Florence, revealed that for many years she'd suspected Diana's mother of secretly using pills, and that this wasn't the first time she'd found her mother passed out. Florence said she'd only later realized that Diana's mother was, in fact, a pill addict. Diana's father would leave Diana every morning with a bottle in her crib on his way out to work at 7:00 am, so that her mother "could sleep." By the time he returned home from work, the house would be neat, and everything looked fine. Florence had been in her early twenties when Diana was a baby, and only appreciated later how insecure, helpless, and self-absorbed Diana's mother had been. At the time, she remembered admiring Diana's mother for seemingly "having her shit together"—a nice husband, a nice house, a baby—while Florence was single, socially awkward, and lonely.

I conducted EMDR[3] sessions with Diana on Florence's reported memory of Diana's childhood neglect. The EMDR processing spurred access to previously dissociated childhood memories of her own, leading her to realize that, despite her proud sense of independence, deep down, she had always carried the belief that she was somehow "not enough." For the first time, her relational patterns were beginning to make sense—"It's been like a continuum of indifference." She then recovered an important childhood memory in which Florence, her mother's best friend, played a key role.

When Diana was four years old, a party had been thrown at her house to welcome her newborn baby sister. She remembered being alone in her room, feeling sad because the baby was getting all the attention. Florence had then arrived at the house. Looking for Diana all over, she'd finally found her alone in her room. Diana remembered seeing Florence standing at her door, holding a toy in her hand that she had brought along with her, just for little Diana.

After recounting this memory, Diana talked about how caring Florence had always been for her, especially in contrast to her own mother's negligence and emotional unpredictability. I noted that Florence had described her youthful impression of Diana's mother ("having her shit together") in exactly the same words Diana had used to describe her own wife when they'd first met, only to discover as time went on, how self-involved and unavailable her wife had become. In her memory, Diana recalled that her mother's best friend Florence, by contrast, would come over and play with Diana as a small child, delighting in her games, and offering her the only focused, undivided attention she had ever known. After this revelation, we were able to work together on how her mother's friend had represented an alternative, more consistent version of maternal attunement. Had Diana somehow unconsciously communicated to me the pain of her longing for emotional attunement, allowing me to energetically pick up the name of the only person in her life by whom she'd ever felt truly nurtured? How ironic, that I'd picked the name "Florence" for her lover, who had initially seemed so exquisitely attuned, only to end up being the opposite of her childhood Florence, and instead replicating her mother's distraction and misattunement, playing out her emotional withdrawal and ultimate rejection.

Diana has since ended her relationship with her lover, deciding she no longer wants to have to work so hard to attain someone else's love. She is focusing on her career and is turning her attention to her own health, family, and to building her own self-regard. I'm not sure how the name "Florence" initially came to me, but ironically the name has come to represent for Diana the consistent nurturing attunement she received from her mother's best friend, rather than the illusive and intoxicating "Florence" of unrequited love.

The synchronicity of my choice of name for Diana's lover, with its complex, dissonant association to Diana's mother's best friend, turned out to be the key that unveiled access to Diana's early childhood trauma of maternal neglect and disorganized attachment, of which Diana had had little conscious memory.

Discussion

How are we to understand these synchronicities, or intuitive manifestations of unconscious entrainment? Had both Diana and Jordan been sending me unconscious "primes," as James Carpenter refers to them in his book *First Sight* (2012)—subtle, unconscious stimuli that guide our perceptions and behaviors outside our conscious awareness? It is possible that Diana was unconsciously cueing me with the childhood longing she felt for her mother's best friend, or that Jordan was unconsciously prompting me to symbolize a way for her to remain connected while also venturing forth to her photography retreat. But even so, how do specific bits of information, such as actual names ("Florence," "Tuckahoe") get transmitted? As scientific research advances, the Newtonian-Cartesian model of the universe is proving increasingly ineffective in answering these questions, so scientists are turning their microscopes further inward looking for answers, toward deeper, subatomic registers. This pursuit has ironically brought quantum theorists to the door of ancient mysticism, aligning with Vedanta and Buddhist concepts such as Goswami's (2008) "universal consciousness," Pauli's "lucid mysticism" (Marin, 2009), or David Bohm's (1980) "implicate order."

When *sensory* "primes" are not available (as with Jordan's telepathic dream of my husband's medical emergency, which took place when we were geographically separated), or when precognitive dreams depict future events (such as my foreknowledge of Sally's presence in New York before running into her later in the subway), it appears that another level of interconnectivity is making itself known. Shapiro and Marks-Tarlow (2021) refer to this as "nonlocal-participatory dynamics" (p. 277). Such theories of nonlocal mind, such as Rupert Sheldrake's (2009) theory of "morphic resonance" (a universal database outside the mind), are still dismissed by mainstream science, as is the increasingly large body of parapsychological research dating back to the nineteenth century. Nonetheless, whether local or nonlocal, these events suggest that a full range of telepathic receptivity might be available to us at all times, manifesting to differing degrees depending upon one's level of emotional need, intentionality, open-mindedness, and variation of conscious awareness of psychic porousness. The continuum model of intuitive responsiveness helps us differentiate between sensory-based, unconscious intuitive communications, and more extreme nonlocal paranormal events that defy the parameters of space and time. If Jordan's telepathic dream represents one extreme of the continuum (since its nonlocality defies space and time), my picking the name "Florence" might be considered a less extreme form of intuitive transmission, since we were both sitting in the same room at the time it occurred, suggesting the possibility of some form of unconscious sensory cue. "Coincidences," synchronicities, or telepathic transmissions like these may occur more often than we realize in clinical work.

One might speculate that some kind of cerebral "filter" or invisible veil gradually developed through human phylogenetic evolution, obscuring paranormal interconnectedness from consciousness in order to preserve the species ("telepathic blindsight," de Peyer, 2016a, 2022). After all, if we all walked around unable to filter out others' feelings, thoughts, sensations, desires, and experiences, we'd be constantly flooded and overwhelmed. Perhaps some of us have greater "leakage" in this "filter" than others, allowing for intuition and telepathic transmissions to pierce the veil protecting our human conscious awareness.

The case of "Diana" illustrates how the appearance of such "leakages" in clinical work can unlock hidden associations, creating openings for therapeutic action when the clinician remains open and receptive. In this case, it was easy for me as the clinician to welcome the telepathic transmission of the name "Florence" with both interest and readiness for exploration, since there was no feeling of personal intrusion or threat. I have no doubt that my uncanny selection of the name "Florence" also resulted in Diana feeling deeply known and understood by me, accelerating our therapeutic work. Without doubt, the intensity of the analytic relationship sets up an emotional substratum that heightens the probability for such occurrences of telepathic transmission to occur. This porousness can be experienced as beneficial or ominous, however, depending on the patient–therapist dynamic and the type of telepathic information transmitted.

Many psychoanalytic accounts of telepathic communication describe the emergence of "psi" when patient (or analyst) is experiencing relational longing, absence, or a sense of loss (Eshel, 2006, 2016). This has certainly been the case in my work with both Jordan and Diana, and many of the uncanny events that I have experienced in my personal life, including my premonition of the boyfriend at the laundromat. Nonetheless, I am reluctant to conflate all paranormal events into one theory. Personal experience, along with a body of research performed by the Stanford Research Institute (Targ & Puthoff, 1974), the Rhine Research Center, established at Duke University in 1935 (Rhine & Pratt, 1957), and the Institute of Noetic Sciences (Radin, 2006), among others, report findings on non-sensory-based forms of transmission such as "remote viewing," psychokinesis, and precognition that all seem to defy the presupposition of relational attachment. With an interest in quantum mechanics, some even speculate that the brain is capable of influencing and receiving "quantum fluctuations" from other brains without direct relational association (Radin, 2003). I am drawn to conclude that a feeling of intense emotional absence or loss is *not always a necessary precursor* for telepathic transmission. My telepathic dream portending Sally's appearance on the subway platform illustrates this, since we had never had a close relationship—in fact, I barely remembered who she was. She held no particular significance for me, and we shared no deep emotional connection or sense of "absence." Uncanny precognitions such as these, which exceed dependency on relational or affective intensity, demonstrate the need to keep an open mind about the greater mystery of paranormal interconnectivity, a mystery that likely cannot be collapsed into any one theoretical framework.

Unbidden and unwilling to be categorized, the paranormal ultimately defies all efforts to be classified or standardized. The mystery of the human psyche, in its agile elusiveness, dodges our control like a dandelion feather in the wind. Perhaps it is time in our field, after one hundred years of skepticism, to surrender to a true state of "evenly hovering attention" by welcoming deep empathic identification, trusting the emergence of spontaneous imagery, and the telepathically informed reverie of a universally shared, creative imagination.

Notes

1 This is often quoted as thus, but, according to Harvard University, the original quote reads: "[W]e with our lives are like islands in the sea, or like trees in the forest. The maple and the pine may whisper to each other with their leaves. But the trees also commingle their roots in the darkness underground, and the islands also hang together through the ocean's bottom. Just so there is a continuum of cosmic consciousness, against which our individuality builds but accidental fences, and into which our several minds plunge as into a mother-sea or reservoir." See https://library.harvard.edu/sites/default/files/static/onlineexhibits/james/psychical/7_8.html

2 "To put it into a formula: [the analyst] must turn his own unconscious like a receptive organ toward the transmitting unconscious of the patient. He must adjust himself to the patient as a telephone receiver is adjusted to the transmitting microphone. Just as the receiver converts back into sound waves the electric oscillations in the telephone line which were set up by sound waves, so the doctor's unconscious is able, from the derivatives of the unconscious which are communicated to him, to reconstruct that unconscious, which has determined the patient's free associations" (pp. 115–116).

3 Eye Movement Desensitization and Reprocessing (EMDR) is a trauma method designed to help patients process traumatic memories.

References

Alcock, J. E. (1998). Science, pseudoscience, and anomaly. *Behavioral and Brain Sciences*, 21, 303–303.

Altman, N. (2002). Where is the action in the "talking cure"? *Contemporary Psychoanalysis*, 38, 499–513.

Aron, L. (1990). One-person and two-person psychologies and the method of psychoanalysis. *Psychoanalytic Psychology*, 7, 475–485.

Baranger, M., & Baranger, W. (2008). The analytic situation as a dynamic field. *International Journal of Psychoanalysis*, 89, 795–826.

Bass, A. (2001). It takes one to know one: Or, whose unconscious is it anyway? *Psychoanalytic Dialogues*, 11, 683–702.

Bays, B. (2014). *The journey: A practical guide to healing your life and setting yourself free*. Atria Books.

Berlin, H. (2011). The neural basis of the dynamic unconscious. *Neuropsychoanalysis*, 13, 5–31.

Beyer, A. C. (2017). Theory of telepathy: An alternative interpretation of psychotic experiences and some tips for recovery. *NeuroQuantology*, 15, 145–159.

Bion, W. R. (1962). *Learning from experience*. Routledge.

Bion, W. R. (1970). *Attention and interpretation*. Basic Books.

Bohm, D. (1980). *Wholeness and the implicate order*. Routledge.

Bollas, C. (1995). *Cracking up: The work of unconscious experience*. Hill & Wang.

Brabant, E., Falzeder, E., & Giampieri-Deutsch, P. (1992). *The correspondence of Sigmund Freud and Sándor Ferenczi*. Belknap Press.

Bromberg, P. M. (2003). One need not be a house to be haunted: On enactment, dissociation, and the dread of "not-me"—A case study. *Psychoanalytic Dialogues*, 13, 689–709.

Cardeña, E., Lynn, S. J., & Krippner, S. (Eds.). (2014). *Varieties of anomalous experience: Examining the scientific evidence* (2nd ed.). American Psychological Association.

Carpenter, J. C. (2012). *First sight: ESP and parapsychology in everyday life.* Rowman & Littlefield.

Carson, S. H., Peterson, J. B., & Higgins, D. M. (2003). Decreased latent inhibition is associated with increased creative achievement in high-functioning individuals. *Personality Processes and Individual Differences*, 85, 499–506.

Civitarese, G., & Ferro, A. (2013). The meaning and use of metaphor in analytic field theory. *Psychoanalytic Inquiry*, 33, 190–209.

de Peyer, J. (2014). Telepathic entanglements: Where are we today? Commentary on paper by Claudie Massicotte. *Psychoanalytic Dialogues*, 24, 109–121.

de Peyer, J. (2016a). Uncanny communication and the porous mind. *Psychoanalytic Dialogues*, 26, 156–174.

de Peyer, J. (2016b). "Presence" and "absence": Kaleidoscopic hide and seek: Reply to commentaries. *Psychoanalytic Dialogues*, 26, 198–205.

de Peyer, J. (2017). Traversing the ineffable: Commentary on Sharon Farber's "Becoming a telepathic tuning fork." *Psychoanalytic Dialogues*, 27, 735–740.

de Peyer, J. (2021). Portals through liminal space: Commentary on Shapiro and Marks-Tarlow's "Varieties of clinical intuition." *Psychoanalytic Dialogues*, 31, 294–301.

de Peyer, J. (2022). Skating on thin ice: Clinical dilemmas with the uncanny. *British Psychological Society, Psychotherapy Section Review*, 67, 62–77.

Eshel, O. (2006). Where are you, my beloved? On absence, loss, and the enigma of telepathic dreams. *International Journal of Psychoanalysis*, 87, 1603–1627.

Eshel, O. (2016). In search of the absent analyst: Commentary on Janine de Peyer's "Uncanny communication." *Psychoanalytic Dialogues*, 26, 185–197.

Ferenczi, S. (1988). *The clinical diary of Sándor Ferenzci* (J. Dupont, Ed.). Harvard University Press. (Original written in 1932).

Frankel, J. (2004). Identification with the aggressor and the "normal traumas": Clinical implications. *International Forum of Psychoanalysis*, 13, 78–83.

Freud, S. (1901). The psychopathology of everyday life: Forgetting, slips of the tongue, bungled actions, superstitions and errors. In J. Strachey (Ed. & Trans.), *The standard edition of the complete psychological works of Sigmund Freud* (Vol. 6, pp. 1–296). Hogarth Press.

Freud, S. (1912). Recommendations to physicians practising psychoanalysis. In J. Strachey (Ed. & Trans.), *The standard edition of the complete psychological works of Sigmund Freud* (Vol. 12, pp. 109–120). Hogarth Press.

Freud, S. (1923). Two encyclopaedia articles. In J. Strachey (Ed. & Trans.), *The standard edition of the complete psychological works of Sigmund Freud* (Vol. 18, pp. 233–260). Hogarth Press.

Freud, S. (1933). New introductory lectures on psychoanalysis. In J. Strachey (Ed. & Trans.) *The standard edition of the complete psychological works of Sigmund Freud* (Vol. 22, pp. 31–56). Hogarth Press.

Gallese, V. (2006). Intentional attunement: Embodied simulation and its role in social cognition. In M. Mancia (Ed.), *Psychoanalysis and neuroscience* (pp. 269–301). Springer.

Gallese, V. (2009). Mirror neurons, embodied simulation, and the neural basis of social identification. *Psychoanalytic Dialogues*, 19, 519–536.

Goswami, A. (2008). *God is not dead: What quantum physics tells us about our origins and how we should live.* Hampton Roads.

Greyson, B. (1977). Telepathy in mental illness: Deluge or delusion? *Journal of Nervous and Mental Disease*, 165, 184–200.

Heisenberg, W. (1927). Ueber den anschaulichen Inhalt der quantentheoretischen Kinematik and Mechanik. *Zeitschrift für Physik*, 43, 172–198.

James, W. (1902). *The varieties of religious experience*. Longmans, Green & Co.

James, W. (1909). The confidences of a "psychical researcher." *American Magazine*, 68, 580–589.

Jung, C. G. (1959). Archetypes of the collective unconscious. In *Collected works of C. G. Jung* (Vol. 9, pp. 3–41). Princeton University Press.

Luckhurst, R. (2023). *The invention of telepathy*. Oxford University Press.

Marin, J. M. (2009). "Mysticism" in quantum mechanics: The forgotten controversy. *European Journal of Physics*, 30, 807–822.

Mascaro, J. S., Rilling, J. K., Negi, L. T., & Raison, C. L. (2013). Compassion meditation enhances empathic accuracy and related neural activity. *Social Cognitive & Affective Neuroscience*, 8, 48–55.

Massicotte, C. (2014). Psychical transmissions: Freud, spiritualism and the occult. *Psychoanalytic Dialogues*, 24, 88–102.

Mayer, E. L. (2001). On "telepathic dreams?" An unpublished paper by Robert J. Stoller. *Journal of the American Psychoanalytic Association*, 49, 629–657.

Mayer, E. L. (2007). *Extraordinary knowing: Science, skepticism, and the inexplicable powers of the human mind*. Bantam Books.

McGilchrist, I. (2009). *The master and his emissary: The divided brain and the making of the western world*. Yale University Press.

Ogden, T. (1997). *Reverie and interpretation: Sensing something human*. Aronson.

Rabeyron, T., Evrard, R., & Massicotte, C. (2020). Psychoanalysis and the sour apple: Thought-transference in historical and contemporary psychoanalysis. *Contemporary Psychoanalysis*, 56, 612–652.

Rabeyron, T., Evrard, R., & Massicotte, C. (2021). Psychoanalysis and telepathic processes. *Journal of the American Psychoanalytic Association*, 69, 535–571.

Radin, D. I. (2003). Thinking about telepathy. *Think*, 1, 23–32.

Radin, D. I. (2006). *Entangled minds*. Paraview Pocket Books.

Radin, D. I. (2013). *Supernormal: Science, yoga, and the evidence for extraordinary psychic abilities*. Random House.

Rhine, J. B. (1934). *Extra-sensory perception* (Vol. 1). Library of Alexandria.

Rhine, J. B., & Pratt, J. G. (1957). *Parapsychology: Frontier science of the mind*. William Morrow.

Rosenbaum, R. (2011). Exploring the other dark continent: Parallels between psi phenomena and the psychotherapeutic process. *The Psychoanalytic Review*, 98, 57–90.

Schore, A. N. (2003). *Affect regulation and the repair of the self*. Norton.

Schwarz, B. E. (1969). Synchronicity and telepathy. *Psychoanalytic Review*, 56, 44–56.

Searles, H. F. (1973). Concerning therapeutic symbiosis. *Annual of Psychoanalysis*, 1, 247–262.

Shapiro, Y., & Marks-Tarlow, T. (2021). Varieties of clinical intuition: Explicit, implicit, and nonlocal neurodynamics. *Psychoanalytic Dialogues*, 31, 262–281.

Sheldrake, R. (2009). *Morphic resonance: The nature of formative causation*. Park Street Press.

Suchet, M. (2004). Whose mind is it anyway? *Studies in Gender and Sexuality*, 5, 259–287.

Targ, R., & Puthoff, H. (1974). Information transmission under conditions of sensory shielding. *Nature*, 251, 602–607.
Tennes, M. (2007). Beyond intersubjectivity: The transpersonal dimension of the psychoanalytic encounter. *Contemporary Psychoanalysis*, 43, 505–525.
Ullman, M. (2003). Dream telepathy: Experimental and clinical findings. In N. Totton (Ed.), *Psychoanalysis and the paranormal: Lands of darkness* (pp. 15–46). Karnac.
Wiseman, R. (1997). *Deception and self-deception: Investigating psychics.* Prometheus Press.
Wiseman, R., & Watt, C. (2004). The illusion of telepathy: A review of the evidence. *Journal of Consciousness Studies*, 11, 1–118.
Winnicott, D. W. (1975). *Through paediatrics to psychoanalysis.* Hogarth Press.

Chapter 4

Discussion of Janine de Peyer's "Piercing the Veil: From Intuition to Telepathic Receptivity"

Richard Reichbart

Richard Reichbart, Ph.D. from the Institute for Psychoanalytic Training and Research (IPTAR) in New York City, comments on Janine De Peyer's paper, noting how her personal experience of a patient in a telepathic dream reproducing an immediate trauma in the analyst's life resembles the reports of other analysts who have had very similar experiences. Experiences taken from a list of patients' telepathic dreams in Richard's 2019 book, The Paranormal Surrounds Us, *include very specific medical issues recounted by the psychoanalysts Robert Stoller and Jule Eisenbud which patients picked up on telepathically. Yet in addition telepathy can also occur when the analyst is experiencing anxiety or embarrassing situations in reality or even in the analyst's own dreams. Richard agrees with Janine that telepathic dreams do not occur only with patients who have experienced loss early in life and are trying unconsciously to remain in contact with the analyst through telepathy, and he believes they occur more generally.*

* * * *

This is a wonderful contribution by Janine de Peyer, so personally revealing of how she was affected by the appearance of telepathic communication with her patient who seemingly accessed the physical crisis of Janine de Peyer's husband, very much as Dr. Eshel was affected by her patient who telepathically accessed Dr. Eshel's attendance at her father's funeral (as she described in the Chapter 1).

But let me emphasize that as wonderful as both presentations are, this type of clinical telepathic data is not newly discovered. Rather—as Renaud Evrard, Julia Gyimesi, and I discuss in chapters that follow—such data have been part of psychoanalysis since the very beginning. The most striking aspect of this for many will be that Janine's patient had a telepathic dream that reflected an immediate traumatic event in Janine's life. This need not always be the case: The patient may pick up on an analyst's thoughts or dreams or experiences that are *not* traumatic but are dynamically invoked for other reasons. Yet the extent to which an immediate traumatic event from the analyst's life can be picked up psychically by the patient is well-documented. Here is only a partial list taken from Chapter 6 of my book *The Paranormal*

DOI: 10.4324/9781003611042-5

Surrounds Us (Reichbart, 2019): A patient dreams of an old man going through a glass door when the analyst Robert Stoller has fallen through a glass door (Mayer, 2001, p. 639); a patient dreams of her teeth on one side of her mouth being broken off at the root when the analyst Robert Stoller's son breaks a tooth in a surfing accident (Mayer, 2001, p. 642); a patient dreams of spilling acid from a box of chemicals that he is pulling in a toy wagon onto his hand and burning it when Robert Stoller's son burned his hand on some chemicals from a toy set (Mayer, 2001, p. 640); a patient dreams of the analyst's daughter having an accident in the snow and being hospitalized when the analyst Jule Eisenbud's daughter has a sledding accident resulting in a broken arm (Eisenbud, 1970, p. 153); or closer to home, a patient dreams of treating a man's exposed intestines the night before the analyst (me) is to go for a colonoscopy the next day (Reichbart, 2019, pp. 151–152). Let me also mention incidents of the analyst's *anxiety* about traumatic events or traumatic thoughts, which a patient may pick up on: A patient dreams of losing two front teeth after the analyst Melanie Suchet dreams of losing two front teeth (Suchet, 2004, p. 273); or—reflecting the kind of associative dynamics that can take place in telepathic communications—a patient anxiously dreams of the analyst Joseph Cambray being lost in the German "Black Forest" on his vacation when the analyst with some trepidation is on his second scuba diving lesson in the Caribbean in an area called the "Black Forest" because of the black coral—a name he did not find out until the very day of the dive (Cambray, 2002, pp. 422–423).

Each psychoanalyst who has experienced telepathic communication in a psychoanalytic session has his or her own story: Ofra Eshel and Janine de Peyer in the previous chapters, and Ruth Rosenbaum, Fonya Helm, and Joao Braga in chapters that follow, have had different experiences of telepathy in psychoanalytic process. Despite our similar experiences, each of us thinks somewhat differently about the phenomena of psi in general. My beliefs are that telepathy is a psi phenomenon that can be particularly important in psychoanalytic process and is the one most likely to occur, but that there is another psi phenomenon—precognition—which does occur (if rarely) in psychoanalytic process, and then there are the phenomena of psychokinesis and apparitions that occur outside. As I indicated in the introduction, my belief came about as a consequence of my first analysis with the psychoanalyst and parapsychologist Jule Eisenbud in Denver over 50 years ago, as well as my experiences living and working with the Navajo Indians as a legal services attorney, and my reading through the years in parapsychology itself, not just psychoanalysis—and of course my work with patients. I have written about my experiences in my book, which is not only about the psychic in Navajo culture and the Navajo understanding of causality, but about the invention of magical sleight of hand by shamans as a way to create a belief system in the audience more likely to induce psi phenomena, and about the extraordinary productions of the psychic photographer Ted Serios with whom my analyst Eisenbud worked, who could project unconscious images on polaroid film. Some of these phenomena are much more difficult to accept, given our cultural biases; they resulted in the psychoanalyst Eisenbud being looked upon as having gone off "the deep end" and being denied Training Analyst status by the New York Psychoanalytic Institute (Pilkington, 1999). Regardless, the extent to which in psychoanalysis we do not educate ourselves about the vast data of psychic phenomena is a travesty. In a sense, I am glad to focus on telepathy in clinical process, because it can be so important and is more easily accepted and provides at least a substantial foot in the psychoanalytic door, so to speak. If we can open the door even a little bit, perhaps eventually we will enter more fully into accepting other manner of psi phenomena.

In this respect, I believe that the data shows that telepathy can occur *frequently* in analytic process. Eisenbud, in his definitive book *Psi and Psychoanalysis: Studies in the Psychoanalysis of Psi-conditioned Behavior* (1970), recounts over 60 telepathic dreams or telepathically registered events of his patients; I recount more than a dozen in my book. My experience is that these psi events tend to come in clusters. Often a patient, in competing for the analyst's attention, will pick up not only on events or dreams of the analyst, but on events or dreams of another patient or patients of the analyst, as if to say as in Freud's Forsyth case (discussed in Chapter 8), "look at me too."

The telepathic dreams or telepathically registered events from my practice, and those of other psychoanalysts through the years, were sometimes of seemingly trivial events and not just traumatic events—almost invariably touching on the lives, dreams, or anxieties of the analyst. I say "seemingly trivial" because often the analyst was experiencing some strong emotion with regard to the underlying event. For example, a patient dreams about company coming to dinner but is concerned that there may not be sufficient silver knives and forks, or there may be a mess, when the analyst worries about whether she has sufficient or good enough cutlery for a dinner party (Pederson-Krag, 1953, pp. 278–279). Or again, a patient dreams of a "chromium soap dish" that he offers to a man, who to his surprise takes it with a smirk when the analyst has taken a chromium soap dish mistakenly shipped to him at the time of construction of his house, which "in a spirit of belligerent dishonesty inspired by rising costs of the house, I had no intention of returning …" (Ullman, 2003, pp. 50–51). Or—a final example—a patient dreams of the analyst in a very loud sport jacket at Atlantic City, looking "Hollywoodish," when the analyst—who has been lobbying his family to go to Atlantic City—to his chagrin bought an unprepossessing sport jacket despite a salesman's suggestion to be bolder (Eisenbud, 1946, pp. 57–59). In addition, there are frequent examples of patients picking up telepathically on what the analyst is reading or what movie the analyst sees. For example, a patient dreams of a bottle of white foam stuff labeled "Appealing Nausea" and of a small leopard the same evening the analyst sees a movie on cats that in an experiment develop an addiction to a mixture of alcohol and milk (Ullman, 2003, p. 19). Or again, an analyst happens to read a recently published psychoanalytic article about an explorer being attacked by a bear, after an analysand compares himself to a bear that will attack the analyst (Reichbart, 2019, pp. 211–212). And then again, there are instances when the analyst and the patient have similar dreams, such as what I previously mentioned: A patient who dreams of losing two front teeth three weeks after the analyst dreams of losing two front teeth (Suchet, 2004, p. 273).

Not surprisingly, since telepathy is part of a paranormal surround that can envelop the psychoanalytic process, it can extend to patients who are being seen by a supervisee, where the patient of the supervisee appears to compete with other patients of the supervising analyst (indicating that this patient too wants attention from the supervisor about whom manifestly the patient does not even know). This is exactly the type of situation that Dr. Braga touches upon in his discussion in Chapter 11 of this book. I offer an example of this in *The Paranormal Surrounds Us* (Reichbart, 2019) in which phallic elements involving an elephant painted red are common to the dreams of two of my patients and at the same time to the patient of my supervisee. And this leads me to something that I feel strongly about, which I have noted in speaking of Freud's principles later on, and that is that telepathy is not like a phone call (even though it may be symbolized in dreams in this way)—it is not a one-way call from the patient to the analyst, which Freud mistakenly believed. Telepathy takes place in a kind of mutuality between psychoanalyst and patient and melds both their unconsciousnesses and their anxieties. This is the point that Janine de Peyer makes so well, which in contrast to Ofra Eshel's experience does not require that the patient have some early childhood trauma or separation. Similarly, as moving and as important as Ofra's data is, I also have no sense that telepathy necessarily occurs as a result of early childhood trauma or separation. It *did* for Ofra's patients, which she elucidates so beautifully and compellingly, but it does not *only* occur with such patients or under these circumstances.

For me, an outstanding question posed by Janine's and Ofra's accounts is: Why do psychoanalysts or people in general in Western culture tend to deny the data of telepathy? I believe that the wonderful at-one-ment experience that Ofra tells of or that Janine implies does not touch upon the overall general resistance to telepathic data in the psychoanalytic community. To illustrate my point, I cite one vignette provided by Dorothy Burlingham (the close companion of Anna Freud). She recounted that a boy threatened his sister with a glass of steaming water shortly after his mother had a rageful thought—of throwing boiling water on someone else (Burlingham, 1953). It was as if the boy, as a consequence of unconscious telepathy, found permission to articulate his own aggression against his sister: "You, mother, wish in anger to throw boiling water on someone, so I can surely do the same to my sister."

Think about what we are saying when someone has a telepathic dream about another person's dream or experience. It is only a very short way to wondering whether a person can be *influenced* in some way by telepathy, not necessarily just by the wonderful at-one-ment of which Ofra speaks, but by the other aspect of psychological functioning of which we as analysts are only too familiar, namely aggression. In 1921, Freud, despite accepting telepathy, observed:

> Perhaps the problem of thought-transference may seem very trivial to you in comparison with the great magical world of the occult. But consider what a momentous step beyond what we have hitherto believed would be involved in this hypothesis alone. What the custodian of [the basilica of] Saint Denis used to add to his account of the saint's martyrdom remains true. Saint Denis is said, after his head was cut off, to have picked it up and to have walked quite a distance with it under his arm. But the custodian used to remark: "In such a case, it is the first step that counts. The rest is easy."
>
> (p. 192)

Ultimately, Freud could not go so far as accepting precognition or psychokinesis, nor I believe does Ofra—the resistance to accepting the psychokinetic data of Ted Serios, who could project images (he never knew exactly what they would be) onto Polaroid camera film with his mind (Eisenbud, 1967), is tremendous for obvious reasons—but the fact is that accepting telepathy in and of itself creates an issue about the possible influence on a person's thinking when it occurs and about aggressive wishes *à la* Saint Denis. The Greek parapsychologist Tanagras (1967) made this point about our resistance to thinking of the possible aggressive aspects of psi, as did Eisenbud (1967), and as do I. Everything that we are taught and which we teach our patients—that wishes are not the same as actions because wishes have no effect in the outside world—gets called into question by the very recognition of telepathy if we let ourselves just wonder about it. We may not want to go there with our patients. We may want to stress with them the important and meaningful connection that telepathy creates, as do Ofra and Janine. And we may want to maintain as best we can the framework of psychoanalysis, which seems generally to work so well—even if in exploring the telepathic connection we do share personal information with our patients that ordinarily we would not—but the fact is that telepathy poses a problem (as surely does psi in general), which we should recognize.

References

Burlingham, D. (1953). Child analysis and the mother (an excerpt). In G. Devereux (Ed.), *Psychoanalysis and the occult* (pp. 188–191). International Universities Press.

Cambray, J. (2002). Synchronicity and emergence. *American Imago*, 59, 409–434.

Eisenbud, J. (1946). Telepathy and problems of psychoanalysis. *Psychoanalytic Quarterly*, 14, 32–87.

Eisenbud, J. (1967). *The world of Ted Serios: "Thoughtographic" studies of an extraordinary mind.* William Morrow & Company.

Eisenbud, J. (1970). *Psi and psychoanalysis: Studies in the psychoanalysis of psi-conditioned behavior.* Grune & Stratton.

Freud, S. (1921). Psychoanalysis and telepathy. In J. Strachey (Ed. & Trans.), *The standard edition of the complete psychological works of Sigmund Freud* (Vol. 18, pp. 177–193). Hogarth Press.

Mayer, E. L. (2001). On "telepathic dreams": An unpublished paper by Robert Stoller. *Journal of the American Psychoanalytic Association*, 49, 639–652.

Pederson-Krag, G. (1953). Telepathy and repression. In G. Devereux (Ed.), *Psychoanalysis and the occult* (pp. 277–287). International Universities Press.

Pilkington, R. (1999) Jule Eisenbud, 1908–1999, a profile in courage. *Journal of Parapsychology*, 63(2). 163–166.

Reichbart, R. (2019). *The paranormal surrounds us: Psychic phenomena in literature, culture and psychoanalysis.* McFarland.

Suchet, M. (2004). Whose mind is it anyway? *Gender and Sexuality*, 5, 259–287.

Tanagras, A. (1967). *Psychophysical elements in parapsychological traditions.* Parapsychology Foundation.

Ullman, M. (2003) Dream telepathy: Experimental and clinical findings. In N. Totton (Ed.), *Psychoanalysis and the paranormal: Lands of darkness* (pp. 15–46). Karnac.

Chapter 5

Parapsychology Explained to Psychoanalysts

A Guide for My Misinformed Colleagues

Renaud Evrard

Renaud Evrard, Ph.D., former President of the Parapsychological Association and former Director of the Institute Metapsyichique International in Paris, is trained in psychoanalytic psychotherapy but unlike the other contributors is not a psychoanalyst. Yet because of his parapsychological background, his chapter is essential reading for any clinician (particularly any psychoanalyst) curious about telepathy in the clinical process. Not only does Renaud briefly summarize the history of telepathy and psychoanalysis (with interesting details), he makes a no-holds-barred plea that psychoanalysts be aware of the scientific data that exists about parapsychology, Parapsychological data has appeared in such mainstream journals as the British Journal of Psychology*;* Science*;* Nature*;* Psychological Bulletin*;* American Psychologist*;* Physics Essays*; and* Frontiers*, and parapsychology is a field of research recognized by the American Association for the Advancement of Science since 1969. Renaud concludes that the failure of establishment psychoanalysis to accept parapsychology represents "a disciplinary isolation, …a scientific cowering, which can only be deleterious to the development of psychoanalysis."*

* * * *

Recent discussions on a psychoanalytic discussion list about parapsychology have triggered some responses, which, although not surprising, always question it. What is the common view, if any, psychoanalysts have regarding parapsychology? A bunch of recent papers have improved the knowledge regarding the history of relations between psychoanalysis and parapsychology (or, mostly, "psychical research," as it was called at the turn of the twentieth century) (Brottman, 2011; Gyimesi, 2016; Massicotte, 2014; Rabeyron et al., 2019, 2020, 2021). Others have dealt with current clinical cases coming from various populations and settings that seem to suggest anomalous cognitions during psychoanalytical therapies (de Peyer, 2014, 2016, 2017; Eshel, 2006, 2010, 2012, 2019; Lazar, 2001; Rosenbaum, 2011; Sànchez-Medina, 2018; Wooffitt, 2017). And a final group of papers develop an analysis of exceptional experiences using a psychoanalytic framework (Rabeyron & Caussié, 2016; Le Maléfan, 2005; Keller et al., 2021; Rabeyron, 2018, 2020; Rabeyron & Bergs, 2020; Si Ahmed,

DOI: 10.4324/9781003611042-6

2014). In this chapter, I will summarize that literature and provide a guide for those who didn't have the time to update their knowledge of this topic.

Where I Am Speaking From

I am not a psychoanalyst myself, but I was trained in France in universities developing an analytical framework and using psychoanalytically inspired psychotherapy in my clinical practice. I developed my interest in the history of psychoanalysis as part of my dissertation thesis on the differential clinical practice with exceptional experiences (ExEs, or so-called paranormal experiences), of which psychoanalysis provides one of the most important clinical paradigms (Si Ahmed, 2014).

Volunteering in organizations promoting parapsychological research, I have held important institutional positions: Director of the Institut Métapsychique International in Paris from 2012 to 2014; and President of the Parapsychological Association from 2019 to 2021, the organization integrated into the American Association for the Advancement of Science since 1969 that brings together most parapsychological researchers. However, I do not consider myself a "parapsychologist," as I have not done any work to prove the existence of an unknown factor such as "psi." My interest is primarily clinical: to help as best I can people struggling with their ExEs, notably within the Center for Information, Research and Counseling on Exceptional Experiences we co-founded with Thomas Rabeyron (now Professor of psychology) in 2009 (Caussié et al., 2016).

I am more in the stream of "metapsychics," as defined by Dr. Hubert Larcher as a disciplinary intersection between psychology, psychopathology, and parapsychology. Dr. Larcher practiced a consultation on ExEs at IMI on a voluntary basis for years (Larcher, 2013), assisted by other clinicians including psychoanalysts such as Juliette Favez-Boutonier.

During my Ph.D., I also worked in an adult psychiatric hospital, before being recruited in 2015 as Assistant Professor of clinical psychology (with a specialty in psychoanalytical psychopathology) at the University of Lorraine, France. All of this is to explain, in a transparent way, that my background has allowed me to build up a first-hand knowledge of the state of scientific parapsychology, although my primary functions are to train future clinical psychologists and to deal with psychological suffering.

Applying Critical Thinking Requires Common Knowledge

I am fully convinced of the value of a critical approach to parapsychology. There is no reason to be enthusiastic about the results obtained after decades of experimental research, nor to hope for the next scientific revolution that will deliver a new ready-made paradigm. I also sometimes despair at the aberrations associated with beliefs and practices claiming to be paranormal. I am therefore also involved in teaching critical thinking and scientific skepticism (sometimes called "zetetic" in French), especially at the University, and I regularly publish critical works on research related to the paranormal (Acunzo et al., 2013; Evrard, 2013).

Institutionally, I am also a member of organizations that promote skepticism (such as the Belgian Committee for the Critical Analysis of Parascience) or anomalistics, that is, a more general and reflexive approach to all empirical claims of anomalies.

I think the common thread in my approach is not to find peers who would support my beliefs, promoting a confirmation bias. I circulate in these different scientific universes in order to collect a maximum of reliable information on the progress of research. It seems obvious to me that debates are richer and more balanced when all parties share a common base of knowledge. Surely everyone must do the same for other fields of interest; nobody would look to debate about psychoanalysis in a cooking class.

So, my goal here is to raise the level of debate by making sure that everyone has access to the same basic information, the "common cultural minimum." Too many differences often lead to polarization of positions, where everyone accuses each other of extremism and incompetence. I absolutely wish that the critical spirit be exercised, even sharpened, and that is why it seems to me necessary that it be based on concrete, verifiable, and shared examples. No one can be at the same time a supporter of a rationality worthy of the Enlightenment (as Freud was) and satisfied to allow the spread of unverified opinions or even lies worthy of obscurantism.

In short, my epistemic attitude is one of humility: I wish to help as best I can those who might disagree with me to show me exactly where I am wrong. Indeed, this would be of greater benefit to me than resting quietly on the feeling that I am right. A static certainty that no longer entails the dynamic exercise of doubt is, in my opinion, the enemy of both the researcher and the clinician, in a psychoanalytic epistemology whose pillars are reflexivity and negative capability (Evrard, 2021).

A Summary of What We Know about the History of Psychoanalysis and Parapsychology

After this preamble to introduce myself and explain my approach, let's move on to a summary of the historical elements that are now widely accepted.

Freud was initially very skeptical about the psychical research of his time. His position evolved until he reached four important conclusions:

- Some parapsychological phenomena are real (mainly thought transference).
- Psychoanalysis and parapsychology are compatible.
- Psychoanalysts should be encouraged to conduct parapsychological research.
- Freud's own career would have been very different if he had been aware earlier of the proven existence of these phenomena and of the possibility of understanding them scientifically.

The factors that favored this evolution are:

- The simultaneous or prior interest of many psychoanalysts in parapsychology (Gyimesi, 2016; Rabeyron & Evrard, 2012).
- Freud's tolerance of this research, which he gradually sought to integrate.
- Freud's own "exploratory" research with mediums and psychics.
- The telepathic occurrences or coincidences collected by Freud in his clinical practice or in his life.
- The reading of the international parapsychological works of his time and the correspondence on this subject with numerous interlocutors.
- Freud's own "experimental" research, which convinced him that he had succeeded in reproducing Gilbert Murray's telepathy protocol (Evrard et al., 2017).

In short, if he positioned psychoanalysis from the outset as an heir to the Enlightenment and as fighting against occultism and a certain number of naive interpretations of phenomena pertaining to psychology, he realized that this position was not incompatible with the existence of phenomena that were awkwardly classified as the rejects of science, even though they were susceptible to scientific study. Freud became a "psychical researcher" (Evrard et al., 2017), whatever one thinks of the quality of his work and ideas on the subject.

On the other hand, several factors were obstacles to this evolution and, more widely, to the public diffusion of this change of attitude:

- Some psychoanalysts had adopted a very critical line towards parapsychology (Evrard & Rabeyron, 2012) .
- The reputation of parapsychology risked discrediting psychoanalysis, if ever the two were associated.
- Freud's exploratory and experimental research was not systematic, and the results were therefore difficult to interpret and were not published.
- Freud's hesitations during his evolution made his positions difficult to read.
- When Freud wished to make his evolution known, notably by adding "The Occult Significance of Dreams" to the final edition of the *Interpretation of Dreams*, he was prevented from doing so by Ernest Jones, then president of the International Psychoanalytical Association (Massicotte, 2014).
- Freud was forced to find a compromise with his own disciples and heirs so that his penchant for parapsychology would appear as one of his whims without compromising the whole discipline he had founded (Jones, 1957).
- Freud's texts on parapsychology (1921, 1922a, 1922b, 1925, 1933) have been belatedly translated, little or poorly commented upon, and, in a way, scotomized.
- Biographers and historians have interpreted this development in various ways, without having recourse to a complete historical record free of the biases linked to black or golden legends.

On the whole, the links between psychoanalysis and parapsychology have gone unnoticed or have been the object of biased interpretations (Jones, 1957), aiming at maintaining the watertightness of the psychoanalytical doctrine in front of its sulfurous neighbor, whose proximity has always been seen as dangerous.

This has not prevented the development of a current of "psychoanalytical parapsychology," of which Georges Devereux's anthology (1953) was the high point; these repressed links between psychoanalysis and parapsychology regularly come back under the pen of more than a hundred authors. Even some non-psychoanalysts like Derrida (1981) could not conceive of a psychoanalysis that would not assimilate telepathy. In the new geopolitics of the psyche, where psychoanalysis is no longer in a hegemonic position in the face of cognitivism and behaviorism, the metapsychist philosopher and sociologist Bertrand Méheust (2006) even called for a change of alliance, opening up to a perennial collaboration between psychoanalysis and parapsychology.

An Introduction to Parapsychology

If these historical elements concerning the history of psychoanalysis have now found their way into the best psychoanalytic journals, the rest of the dossier still struggles to be heard or read. Indeed, we can find another literature that focuses on telepathic-like phenomena or coincidences occurring during psychoanalytic cures (de Peyer, 2014, 2016, 2017; Eshel, 2006, 2010, 2012, 2019; Lazar, 2001; Rosenbaum, 2011; Sànchez-Medina, 2018; Wooffitt, 2017), or the application of psychoanalysis to the understanding and treatment of ExEs (Le Maléfan, 2005; Keller et al., 2021; Rabeyron, 2018, 2020; Rabeyron & Bergs, 2020; Rabeyron & Caussié, 2016; Si Ahmed, 2014). Some of these publications are already adventurous, slipping in references relating to experimental parapsychology, or concerning theoretical models, more or less faithful to quantum physics, likely to increase the intelligibility of the whole.

More rarely, we find echoes of psychoanalysts experiencing themselves, outside the treatment, ostensibly "paranormal" phenomena, such as the episode of clairvoyance experienced by Mayer (2007). But there are also psychoanalysts who have taken the step of experimental research and have become openly "parapsychologists," such as Nandor Fodor, Emilio Servadio, Jule Eisenbud (1966), Jan Ehrenwald, or even Montague Ullman, the latter even becoming president of the Parapsychological Association in 1966.

Having submitted several articles relating to the history and current status of the problem of telepathy in psychoanalysis, I have experienced some quite fabulous peer reviews where, beyond the expression of hostility and ignorance, a paradoxical request was made: Either the authors of the article had to publish a state of the art of parapsychological research, or they had to elide absolutely the hypothesis of a possible reality of telepathy or psi. This double bind often led to a dead end, because an article synthesizing parapsychological research does not really belong in a psychoanalytic journal, the proof being that no psychoanalytic journal has published such an article, whereas one can find them in many psychological and physical journals (see below). The alternative of never melding the parapsychological approach with the psychoanalytical approach could only result in the maintenance of a dogmatic attitude that cuts off any possibility of scientifically exploring certain clinical materials.

Why do these reviewers, whom I consider to be my colleagues, encourage ignorance? The reality is probably different, since it is possible to talk about parapsychology in the interstices of psychoanalytical congresses, in the privacy of one's own home, while explicitly or implicitly revering the taboo in the official approach to "psychoanalytical parapsychology." This could still be justified if it were an attitude that was not specific to the psychoanalytic movement. But my impression is that, by doing so, this movement is further distancing itself from the scientific consensus, which is progressively moving towards an increased recognition of the scientific quality of parapsychology, of the value of its results, and of the fruitfulness of its theoretical proposals (Cardeña et al., 2015).

The misnamed "parapsychology" is a scientific discipline that became institutionalized from the 1880s, in the form of the first psychological societies (Evrard, 2016). After the study of extraordinary performances of rare, gifted subjects, it focused from the 1930s on the systematic study of micro-phenomena more easily reproducible in average individuals. Experimental methodology and statistical analysis became its main modus operandi. Nevertheless, research has increasingly integrated elements from the human sciences. An example is the series of research on telepathic dreaming initiated by psychoanalyst Ullman and psychologist Stanley Krippner (Ullman et al., 1973), where dream narratives were compared with images, one of which was the randomly selected target while the others were decoys. This allowed for a dual analysis: quantitative with judgments matching the stories with the correct targets; and qualitative with analysis of dream symbolism and associations of ideas showing how the target had been accommodated in the dreamer's mind.

Parapsychology became an academic discipline in 1912 at Stanford. In the 1980s, the center of gravity of the research shifted back to Europe. Dozens of universities now have research and teaching units in parapsychology or anomalistic psychology. In total, 43 universities worldwide offer courses or training at the Master's level in parapsychology or anomalistic psychology (Zingrone, 2011).

In this academic environment, parapsychology has somewhat "mutated." It is now presented more as a specialty of psychology known as anomalistic psychology. It examines so-called paranormal beliefs and experiences in order to explain them by known or yet to be discovered psychological hypotheses. It is a more mono-disciplinary view than parapsychology, with a reference work, the *Varieties of Anomalous Experience* (Cardeña et al., 2014), published by the American Psychological Association, which is in its second edition.

Anomalistic psychology and parapsychology now have numerous textbooks used in university teaching (Holt et al., 2012; Irwin & Watt, 2007; Roe & Sherwood, 2011).

Currently, six specialized journals regularly publish quality articles: *Journal of the Society for Psychical Research*; *Journal of Anomalistics*; *Journal of Scientific Exploration*; *Journal of Parapsychology*; *Australian Journal of Parapsychology*; and the *Journal of Anomalous Experience and Cognition.*

Do parapsychologists only practice the "*entre-soi*"? One need only look around to see that parapsychologists actually publish in every scholarly journal, from every discipline, and have done so for decades. Dean Radin maintains a web page[1] with the main publications on experimental evidence in parapsychology, on which one can notice that they are distributed in so-called "mainstream" journals or others more specialized: *British Journal of Psychology*; *Science*; *Nature*; *Psychological Bulletin*; *American Psychologist*; *Physics Essays*; *Frontiers*, and so on.

Together with my late German colleague Gerd Hövelmann and my Dutch colleague Maurice van Luijtelaar, we have been collecting relevant articles on the paranormal in mainstream journals since 2009. In the columns of *Mindfield*, the bulletin of the Parapsychological Association, we have listed a total of 2,691 publications, which is about 200 per year or 4 per week. As all disciplines are concerned, from psychology to physics to literature, no researcher is in fact able to fully absorb what is happening in this transdisciplinary field.

This observation leads me to say that any claim to be familiar with the parapsychological literature is audacious. The transdisciplinary skills needed to decipher certain articles are indeed very demanding. Add to this an equal knowledge of the so-called skeptical literature, and it becomes extremely rare indeed to be able to overlook this discipline.

In January 2018, *American Psychologist*, one of the most important psychology journals, published a particularly favorable review of the experimental evidence for parapsychological phenomena. Its sole author is Etzel Cardeña, a professor of psychology of Mexican origin, who holds the Thorsen Chair of Hypnosis and Parapsychology at Lund University in Sweden, the oldest university in that country.

In his article, Cardeña makes a clear and concise presentation of what parapsychology is, summarizes some of the theories that make "psi phenomena" intelligible, before providing an overview of the experimental results. Let's proceed to his conclusion, which is not lacking in piquancy in such a context: He considers that the accumulated evidence supports the reality of "psi" and cannot be explained by poor quality studies, fraud, selective publication of only the successful ones, incompetence in experimental methodology or analysis, or by other frequent criticisms. In the end, Cardeña leaves the skeptical reader with no way out, crushed under the weight of the "facts."

In his comparisons with other scientific disciplines, especially psychology, he shows that the level of evidence attained by parapsychologists is on a par with other phenomena considered firmly established. However, the problem lies in the interpretation of these phenomena, which is far from having reached any consensus. Cardeña nevertheless makes some recommendations in order to further secure our confidence in these results, while developing tests specifically aimed at selecting the best theoretical model.

In Cardeña's article, Table 1 summarizes the meta-analytic results for the six paradigms testing anomalous cognition: the Ganzfeld; precognition studies in the line of the social psychologist Darryl Bem; studies employing dreaming; remote viewing; presentiment; and forced choice precognition. All of these experimental paradigms have obtained statistically significant results in thousands of trials over decades of research.

Cardeña also examines anomalous disturbances whose effects are detected by statistical analysis. He dismisses from his review the study of "anomalous forces" that would be measured by other means, such as a measurement of mechanical deformation in the case of thought-twisted metal bars. Some studies focus on intentional effort to change a parameter—such as concentration—of a remote living system. This effort may take the form of attempted healing ("remote healing"), visual observation ("remote staring"), or support ("remote helping"). Table 2 synthesizes the results of these three neighboring research paradigms on remote influence, each with significantly positive cumulative results.

Thus, the official journal of the American Psychological Association, the most important psychological society in the world, published an article stating that the level of evidence in parapsychology has reached the bar set by the scientific community. For decades, researchers have been obtaining results that the majority of Westerners consider impossible. By dint of perseverance, they have managed to confirm that their quest was not totally in vain. Cardeña points out that the affirmation of the existence of psi is supported both vertically, in the sense that these different protocols have continued to produce results for decades, beyond what we could expect from chance, with a constantly improving methodological rigor; and horizontally, in the sense that psi seems to have manifested itself in different research fields (Cardeña et al., 2015). To put it in a way that is as realistic as it is provocative, there has been more progress in the experimental approach to psi phenomena—and probably in their demonstration—than to the processes described by the different schools of psychoanalysis.

But why study these phenomena if they are impossible? This is, at present, the main answer to Cardeña's article, published in the same prestigious journal. As staggering as it may seem, the skeptical psychologists Arthur Reber and James Alcock (2020) have indeed elaborated a line of defense against the parapsychological tsunami worthy of the greatest dogmas of the Middle Ages. One of their formulas sums up their argument well: "the data are irrelevant" (Reber & Alcock, 2019). In other words, nothing can change their minds.

Imagine for a moment a scientist saying that there is no point in conducting laboratory experiments, analyzing their results, and compiling the data obtained by independent researchers around the world. Imagine this scientist defending an anti-empirical approach to science by arguing: We have theories that work well, why should we change them?

This position seems like a radical turn: Don't skeptics usually profess that parapsychological experiments have failed? To consider that it is rationally possible to be indifferent to their success would be to fall into an assumed form of denial. Finally, to reach such an extreme argument risks a backlash, since such a position is untenable in the long run and totally contrary to the conventional positions of scholars.

Conclusion: Some Arguments Psychoanalysts Should Be Wary of

I do not imagine that the psychoanalytic movement will evolve overnight, devoting sessions of congresses to psychoanalytic parapsychology, usually welcoming articles on these aspects in their journals, and the like. It took Freud nearly 20 years to make this journey, after having already shown his epistemic mobility by moving from neurology to hypnotherapy, and then from hypnotherapy to a whole new method.

For all that, I cannot conceive that my psychoanalytic colleagues maintain anachronistic positions, without updating their knowledge at least. To find again and again the same arguments about the absence of experimental evidence, the danger to the public, the scientific marginality, the amalgam with occultism and mysticism, the lack of relevance, the adherence to pseudo-skeptical demystifications … seems to me to be the sign of a disciplinary isolation, of a scientific cowering, which can only be deleterious to the development of psychoanalysis. We should not follow the example of the Catholic Church in its relationship to the theory of evolution. Freud showed us, true to his commitments, that epistemic courage was a cardinal virtue of his approach, even if this does not mean that this is a sure way to reach the truth.

Certainly, parapsychology is not a totally established science, it would be more accurate to speak of it as a proto-science, which, at its best, offers all the guarantees of an adequate application of scientific methodology (French & Stone, 2013). But this discipline was structured a little before psychoanalysis by playing a very influential role in the first dynamic psychiatry (Ellenberger, 1970). It is time to reconsider some of the Enlightenment-labeled judgments that cast opprobrium on experiences and phenomena that are so important to human beings. And if there is to be a psychoanalytic critique of parapsychological research, it can only be applied concretely to data that have been constantly accumulated and refined for more than a century. Freud (1966) stated that if he could return to the beginning of his career, he would devote himself to parapsychology. Rather than dismissing this encounter with such idealistic regret, we have the opportunity to foster an intellectual convergence that will certainly benefit both worlds.

Note

1 See https://www.deanradin.com/recommended-references?fbclid=IwAR2gWLXtSBYkoPhVoSG7ePPTBFR-2BRRyOcXBjy9PVuwZu_-UUYVG4HkmIo

References

Acunzo, D. J., Evrard, R., & Rabeyron, T. (2013). Anomalous experiences, psi, and functional neuroimaging. *Frontiers in Human Neuroscience*, 7, 893.

Brottman, M. (2011). *Phantoms of the clinic: From thought-transference to projective identification*. Karnac.

Cardeña, E., Lynn, S. J., & Krippner, S. (Eds.) (2014). *Varieties of anomalous experiences: Examining the scientific evidence* (2nd ed.). American Psychological Association.

Cardeña, E., Palmer, J., & Marcusson-Clavertz, D. (Eds.) (2015). *Parapsychology: A handbook for the 21st century*. McFarland.

Caussié, S., Charlet, O., Evrard, R., & Rabeyron, T. (2016). Introducing CIRCEE. *Journal of Exceptional Experiences and Psychology*, 4, 12–14.

de Peyer, J. (2014). Telepathic entanglements: Where are we today? Commentary on paper by Claudie Massicotte. *Psychoanalytic Dialogues*, 24, 109–121.

de Peyer, J. (2016). Uncanny communication and the porous mind. *Psychoanalytic Dialogues*, 26, 156–174.

de Peyer, J. (2017). Traversing the ineffable: Commentary on Sharon Farber's "Becoming a telepathic tuning fork." *Psychoanalytic Dialogues*, 27, 735–740.

Derrida, J. (1981). Télépathie. *Cahiers confrontations*, 10, 201–230.

Devereux, G. (Ed.). (1953). *Psychoanalysis and the occult*. International Universities Press.

Eisenbud, J. (1966). *The world of Ted Serios: "Thoughtographic" studies of an extraordinary mind*. William Morrow.

Ellenberger, H. F. (1970). *The discovery of the unconscious: The history and evolution of dynamic psychiatry*. Basic Books.

Eshel, O. (2006). Where are you, my beloved? On absence, loss, and the enigma of telepathic dreams. *International Journal of Psychoanalysis*, 87, 1603–1627.

Eshel, O. (2010). Patient-analyst interconnectedness: Personal notes on close encounters of a new dimension. *Psychoanalytic Inquiry*, 30, 146–154.

Eshel, O. (2012). A beam of "chimeric" darkness: Presence, interconnectedness, and transformation in the psychoanalytic treatment of a patient convicted of sex offenses. *Psychoanalytic Review*, 99, 149–178.

Eshel, O. (2019). Would clinical psychoanalysis shy away from delving further into the unknown? On the mystery of telepathic dreams. *International Journal of Psychoanalysis*, 100, 608–610.

Evrard, R. (2013). Répercussions psychologiques des "souvenirs" de la mort propre: Une critique des travaux du Dr Pim van Lommel. *Etudes sur la mort*, 143, 159–172.

Evrard, R. (2016). *La légende de l'esprit: Enquête sur 150 ans de parapsychologie*. Trajectoire.

Evrard, R. (2021). Trois piliers de l'esprit scientifique: Contributions psychanalytiques à une méta-théorie de la connaissance. *Psychologues & Psychologies*, 275, 45–54, doi:10.3917/pep.275.0003g.

Evrard, R., Massicotte, C., & Rabeyron, T. (2017). Freud as a psychical researcher: The impossible Freudian legacy. *Imágó Budapest*, 6, 9–32.

Evrard, R., & Rabeyron, T. (2012). Les psychanalystes et le transfert de pensée: Enjeux historiques et actuels. *L'Evolution Psychiatrique*, 77, 589–598.

French, C. C., & Stone, A. (2013). *Anomalistic psychology: Exploring paranormal belief and experience*. Palgrave Macmillan.

Freud, S. (1921). Psychoanalysis and telepathy. In G. Devereux (Ed.), *Psychoanalysis and the occult* (pp. 56–68). International Universities Press.

Freud, S. (1922a). Dreams and telepathy. In G. Devereux (Ed.), *Psychoanalysis and the occult* (pp. 69–86). International Universities Press.

Freud, S. (1922b). Some neurotic mechanisms in jealousy, paranoia and homosexuality. In J. Strachey (Ed. & Trans), *The standard edition of the complete psychological works of Sigmund Freud* (Vol. 18, pp. 223–232). Hogarth Press.

Freud, S. (1925). The occult significance of dreams. In G. Devereux (Ed.), *Psychoanalysis and the occult* (pp. 87–90). International Universities Press.

Freud, S. (1933). Dreams and the occult. In G. Devereux (Ed.), *Psychoanalysis and the occult* (pp. 91–109). International Universities Press.

Freud, S. (1966). *Correspondence, 1873–1939*. Gallimard.

Gyimesi, J. (2016). Why "spiritism"? *International Journal of Psychoanalysis*, 97, 357–383.

Holt, N., Simmonds-Moore, C., Luke, D., & French, C. (2012). *Anomalistic psychology*. Palgrave Macmillan.

Irwin, H. J., & Watt, C. (2007). *An introduction to parapsychology* (5th ed.). McFarland.

Jones, E. (1957). *The life and work of Sigmund Freud (Vol. 3): The last phase, 1919–1939*. Hogarth Press.

Keller, L., Szymkiewicz, A., Mutis, M., & Evrard, R. (2021). Complaisance du hasard et expériences de coïncidences. *L'Evolution Psychiatrique*, 86, 285–306.

Larcher, H. (2013). *L'odyssée de la conscience: Anthologie d'études sur la mort, la mystique et le paranormal par le Dr Hubert Larcher*. Editions de l'Institut Métapsychique International.

Lazar, S. G. (2001). Knowing, influencing, and healing: Paranormal phenomena and implications for psychoanalysis and psychotherapy. *Psychoanalytic Inquiry*, 21, 113–131.

Le Maléfan, P. (2005). La "sortie hors du corps" est-elle pensable par nos modèles cliniques et psychopathologiques? Essai de clinique d'une marge. À propos d'un cas. *L'Evolution Psychiatrique*, 70, 513–534.

Massicotte, C. (2014). Psychical transmissions: Freud, spiritualism, and the occult. *Psychoanalytic Dialogues*, 24, 88–102.

Mayer, E. L. (2007). *Extraordinary knowing: Science, skepticism, and the inexplicable powers of the human mind*. Bantam Dell.

Méheust, B. (2006). Le dégoût et l'effroi: La nécessité d'un changement d'alliance. In T. Nathan (Ed.), *La guerre des psys: Manifeste pour une psychothérapie démocratique* (pp. 123–150). Les Empêcheurs de Penser en Rond.

Rabeyron, T. (2018). Clinique des expériences d'abduction: Trauma, clivage et logiques de l'originaire. *L'Evolution Psychiatrique*, 83, 355–379.

Rabeyron, T. (2020). *Clinique des expériences exceptionnelles*. Dunod.

Rabeyron, T., & Bergs, A. (2020). Clinique des expériences de mort imminente: Du vécu agonistique aux formes extrêmes de symbolisation. *L'Evolution Psychiatrique*, 85, 407–426.

Rabeyron, T., & Caussié, S. (2016). Clinical aspects of out-of-body experiences: Trauma, reflexivity and symbolization. *L'Évolution Psychiatrique*, 81, e53-e71.

Rabeyron, T., & Evrard, R. (2012). Historical and contemporary perspectives on occultism in the Freud-Ferenczi correspondence. *Research in Psychoanalysis*, 13, 98–111.

Rabeyron, T., Evrard, R., & Massicotte, C. (2019). "Es gibt Gedankenübertragung": Transfert de pensée et processus télépathiques en analyse. *Revue Française de Psychanalyse*, 83, 1239–1252.

Rabeyron, T., Evrard, R., & Massicotte, C. (2020). Psychoanalysts and the sour apple: Thought-transference in historical and contemporary psychoanalysis. *Contemporary Psychoanalysis*, 56, 612–652.

Rabeyron, T., Evrard, R., & Massicotte, C. (2021). Psychoanalysis and telepathic processes. *Journal of the American Psychoanalytic Association*, 69, 535–571.

Reber, A. S., & Alcock, J. E. (2019). Why parapsychological claims cannot be true. *Skeptical Inquirer*, 3, 8–10.

Reber, A. S., & Alcock, J. E. (2020). Searching for the impossible: Parapsychology's elusive quest. *American Psychologist*, 75, 391–399.

Roe, C. A., & Sherwood, S. (2011). *Anomalistic psychology*. Palgrave Macmillan.

Rosenbaum, R. (2011). Exploring the other dark continent: Parallels between psi phenomena and the psychotherapeutic process. *Psychoanalytic Review*, 98, 57–90.

Sànchez-Medina, A. (2018). Projective identification and "telepathic dreams". *International Journal of Psychoanalysis*, 99, 380–390.

Si Ahmed, D. (2014). *Pour une psychanalyse des expériences exceptionnelles: Comment penser le paranormal*. L'Harmattan.

Ullman, M., Krippner, S., & Vaughan, A. (1973). *Dream telepathy*. Hampton Roads Publishing.

Wooffitt, R. (2017). Relational psychoanalysis and anomalous communication: Continuities and discontinuities in psychoanalysis and telepathy. *History of the Human Sciences*, 30, 118–137.

Zingrone, N. (2011). Petition to submit a proposal for a Masters of Arts in parapsychology. Unpublished document. Atlantic University.

Chapter 6

Sándor Ferenczi and the Problem of Telepathy[1]

Júlia Gyimesi

It is only fitting that our group of psychoanalysts—from different countries and psychoanalytic orientations—has a contribution from the Hungarian psychoanalyst Júlia Gyimesi, Ph.D. Here Júlia recounts in rich detail how the famed Hungarian psychoanalyst Ferenczi, companion to Freud, believed in and approached the phenomenon of telepathy in clinical process. As with the subsequent lack of recognition of Freud's work on telepathy, Ferenczi's interest in and exploration of telepathy have tended to be minimized by contemporary psychoanalysis.

* * * *

It is well known that Sándor Ferenczi, the great representative of the Budapest School of Psychoanalysis, was a real innovator. His contributions to the technique and theory of psychoanalysis proved to be fundamental in its history. It is less known that Ferenczi was also influenced by psychical research and spiritualism. Although it is not easy to estimate the effects of his telepathy experiments in light of his innovations, it is unquestionable that Ferenczi was deeply interested in thought-transference and encouraged systematic research in the field.

Ferenczi was not alone among psychoanalysts in his interest in psychical research and spiritualism. The founder of psychoanalysis, Sigmund Freud, was also deeply involved in the question of telepathy and made some remarkable observations on the phenomena (Freud, 1904, 1921, 1922, 1933). In his opinion, telepathy was a psychoanalytically significant question that could illuminate the physical equivalents of mental processes. Carl Gustav Jung, Freud's heretical disciple, was labeled as a mystic, since in his analytical psychology he integrated the theory of psychoanalysis with spiritualism, religion, astrology, alchemy, and Eastern philosophies (Jung, 1896, 1897, 1902, 2009). He was also truly interested in psychical research and parapsychology; he conducted several experiments with mediums and published numerous articles on the connection between the functioning of the unconscious and parapsychology (Jung, 1933, 1944, 1977). Many other representatives of early psychoanalysis were also interested in psychical research; István Hollós[2] (1933), Helene Deutsch (1926), John Rickman (1933), and T. W. Mitchell

DOI: 10.4324/9781003611042-7

(1918, 1938) are only some of those who tried to interpret the spiritualistic and other seemingly supernatural phenomena in psychoanalytic terms. As a result of their efforts, valuable psychoanalytic theories were born, which enriched the understanding of human relationships with innovative ideas. Their main interest remained thought-transference, which they declared relevant in the interpretation of the psychoanalytic situation.

Other psychoanalysts, like Freud's biographer Ernest Jones (1931, 1957), were also certainly involved in the question of supernatural phenomena; however, their primary aim was to disprove the validity of such phenomena and identify the psychoanalytic, rationalistic meaning of supernatural belief systems. In their theories they followed a skeptical, reductive method of interpretation in which the seemingly supernatural phenomena were debunked by psychoanalytic theories; therefore, they conformed to the demands of medical materialism.

In one way or another, psychoanalysts were deeply involved in the question of the supernatural. Partly as a result of this, historians of psychology often identify psychoanalysis with a mystical, irrational approach, which is rather far from the realm of science. They usually ignore the fact that psychoanalysts had very different attitudes towards the so-called "occult," and most of them pursued an objective and rational method of understanding in their theories. Furthermore, psychoanalysts were not more involved in the question of spiritualistic phenomena or psychical research than the representatives of other branches of psychology. Their interest in these occurrences was a typical feature of early psychological thinking, in which mediumistic performances and other inexplicable phenomena seemed to be an excellent field for psychological investigations. By researching the latter, psychologists developed many different theories on the possible psychological background of mediumism. Among these, the theory of subliminal or unconscious processes proved to be fundamental; therefore, it is not surprising that numerous psychoanalysts started to focus on the field of supernatural phenomena.

As has been pointed out (Luckhurst, 2002; Oppenheim, 1988; Treitel, 2004), the scientific investigation of mediumistic and spiritualistic phenomena developed in connection with the discoveries and changes of nineteenth-century science and culture. The most important organization in these researches was the Society for Psychical Research (SPR), founded in London in 1882. The representatives of the SPR encouraged systematic investigation in the field of hypnotism, mesmerism, spiritualistic and psychical phenomena, and as a result of their efforts, valuable theories were born on the possible psychological and physical background of the seemingly supernatural occurrences. Among these, Frederic Myers' concept on the subliminal consciousness also proved to be highly significant for the psychoanalysts. Freud was aware of Myers' theory and—although there were some potential links between his own theory of the unconscious and the subliminal self—he tried to distance himself from the realm of Myersian subliminal psychology (Freud, 1912; Hinshelwood, 1995; Keeley, 2001). Freud insisted on the materialist origins of the human psyche, and despite the fact that he was interested in psychical research, at heart he was rather ambivalent and cautious about the results of psychical researchers. However, Freud's efforts to demarcate psychoanalysis from Myers' concept of the subliminal self played an extraordinary role in the systematic theorization of the Freudian concept of unconscious.

Ferenczi was one of those psychoanalysts who did not intend to disprove the validity of apparently supernatural phenomena. Nevertheless, in his technical and theoretical innovations—according to which the psychoanalyst was an active, emotionally, and intuitively accessible actor in the psychoanalytic situation (Ferenczi, 1928, 1932a, 1932b)—he seemingly ignored the results of his experiments with telepathy. Taking into account the significance of Ferenczi's theories for the later development of psychoanalysis, it would be misleading to neglect the influence of his experiments and ideas in the field of spiritualism and psychical research. Although he never developed a comprehensive theory on the matter, his interest in apparently supernatural phenomena was a typical manifestation of his innovative attitude, which proved to be so fruitful in psychoanalysis. Therefore, it is worth examining whether his interest in the abovementioned phenomena might have influenced the development of his ideas and technical considerations. In this chapter, I will argue that although Ferenczi's theories on telepathy were not elaborated, they developed in connection with his most significant innovations and thus they influenced Ferenczi's ideas in a significant way.

Ferenczi discusses spiritualism in one of his earliest publications, in 1899. The fact that he devoted one of his first writings to the subject of spiritualism says a lot about the openness of the young Ferenczi. It reveals not only his scientific attitudes, but the innovative enthusiasm which characterized so many scientists at the turn of the last century. William James, Théodore Flournoy, Carl Gustav Jung, Charles Richet, and Frederic Myers are only some of those eminent scholars who encouraged systematic investigation in the field of spiritualistic phenomena and thus enriched early psychology with valuable results (see Flournoy, 1900; James, 1886; Jung, 1902; Myers, 1903; Richet, 1923). Besides American, English, French, and German psychology, Hungarian scientific life was also influenced by spiritualism (Elekes, 1926; Szántó, 1927; Szilágyi, 1923), although psychical research was not so well known and widespread in Hungary. Instead of the unorganized nature of psychical research in Hungary, Ferenczi followed the objectivity of psychical researchers in his early investigations in the field of spiritualism.

Nevertheless, Ferenczi's publication on spiritism (1899) raises many questions. What is the significance of this early article in Ferenczi's life work? Was his interest in spiritualistic phenomena determining, or was it only a transitory enthusiasm? Why did Ferenczi devote an article to spiritualism in the first years of his psychological career? What is the connection between this article and his later psychoanalytic theories? The aim of the present chapter is to try to answer these questions.

On Spiritism

Ferenczi was not the only one in the history of psychoanalysis who started his scientific career with a publication on spiritualistic phenomena.[3] In 1902, Carl

Gustav Jung published his doctoral dissertation "On the Psychology and Pathology of So-called Occult Phenomena," in which he examined the special abilities of S. W., a young female medium. In reality, S. W. was his cousin, Helene Preiswerk, whose mediumistic trance-states were interpreted using Jung's theory of hysteria and somnambulism (Jaffé, 1971; Zumstein-Preiswerk, 1975). His work bears witness to a typical way of thinking of the early representatives of psychoanalysis and psychology, in which the psychological interpretation of mediumistic performances concluded with the postulation of unconscious processes and automatisms.

Similarly to Jung, Ferenczi attributed special psychological significance to the subject of spiritualistic phenomena. In his article "Spiritism" (1899), he encouraged systematic investigations in the field of spiritualism:

> Therefore the antagonists of spiritism should not use denial before, or without investigation in their crusade. They should devote themselves to the investigation of the claimed facts with the same objectivity that characterizes science in other fields. They should not shrink from sitting down at the moving table or from visiting spiritistic gatherings of lay people. After all, from the sociological point of view alone, the subject is important enough to attract the attention of the best minds. Let them take with themselves the arsenal of science, let them organize experimental seances, observe, rule out intentional deception and decide how much is delusion and how much is truth.
>
> Even though their findings may not establish the objectivity of spiritualistic claims, subjective findings of truth would certainly be made.
>
> (p. 143)

As did many of his other contemporaries, Ferenczi supposed that spiritualistic phenomena were based on the split of psychological functions or automatisms (Janet, 1930; Jung, 1902). Therefore, they refer to a hidden, subconscious functioning of the psyche, which could have exceptionally important scientific significance. Although his views on the subject are rather general and introductory, they reflect the main interests of the young Ferenczi: the border zones of science and the automatic or unconscious functioning of the psyche.

It is worth mentioning that his article on "Spiritism" was the result of Ferenczi's openness to accept the reality of spiritualistic phenomena: In the early years of his career, he conducted several experiments with automatic writing. It was the "pencil's idea" to write an article on spiritualism and send it to Miksa Schächter, who was the editor of a well-known Hungarian medical journal, *Gyógyászat* (Ferenczi, 1917). The fact that Ferenczi followed the advice of the pencil proves that he was not skeptical towards spiritualistic occurrences, although a kind of playfulness characterized him. The abovementioned experiments with automatic writing were not the only sign of Ferenczi's interest in spiritualism; he published valuable reviews on issues of psychical research (Ferenczi, 1900a, 1900b). As his later works illuminate, Ferenczi was obviously not a spiritualist, but to a certain degree he was open to accepting the non-materialistic reality of spiritualistic phenomena, which he tried to interpret with psychological concepts.

Telepathy Experiments

Although Ferenczi was not an active member of the Society for Psychical Research (he was an associate of the society from 1911), in his psychoanalytic practice, he conducted several experiments with mediums and clairvoyants. In these investigations, he followed the objectivity of psychical researchers, trying to find a scientific interpretation for the phenomena (see Brabant et al., 1993). His enthusiasm was a determining factor in his telepathy experiments from the beginning, and, as a result, he never gave up seeking evidence concerning the reality of the seemingly supernatural phenomena. His primary aim was to convince skeptical others, especially Freud, of the existence of telepathy; their correspondence bears witness to his efforts.

In his letters, Ferenczi regularly gave accounts of his results, and it seems that Freud—in spite of his skepticism—was almost as interested in the question as his disciple. However, Freud tried to hold Ferenczi back from publishing the results of his experiments. He was worrying about the consequences of such a publication concerning the often-questioned scientific image of psychoanalysis. In the scientific legitimation of psychoanalysis, its materialist principles, especially the theory of sexuality, played an extraordinary role, due to which—instead of the critiques and the attacks on psychoanalysis—the Freudian theory could become a part of science. Freud was aware of the special significance of the theory of sexuality. It was Jung (1961) himself who summarized the role that Freud intended to give to it:

> I can still recall vividly how Freud said to me, "My dear Jung, promise me never to abandon the sexual theory. That is the most essential thing of all. You see we must make a dogma of it, an unshakable bulwark." He said that to me with great emotion, in the tone of a father saying, "And promise me this one thing, my dear son: that you will go to church every Sunday." In some astonishment I asked him, "A bulwark—against what?" To which he replied, "Against the black tide of mud"—and here he hesitated for a moment, then added—"of occultism."
>
> (p. 173)

Thus, the theory of sexuality guaranteed the scientific nature of psychoanalysis and protected it from the suspicion of occultism.

It must be added that Freud was not so cautious in the case of his own observations on the subject of telepathy; during his career he wrote numerous articles and lectures on the problem (see Devereux, 1953). Despite the efforts of his biographer, Ernest Jones (1957), Freud was rather open to connecting psychoanalysis with the question of telepathy, but in doing so, he always focused on the psychoanalytic and not the spiritualistic significance of the phenomena.

However, Freud's aim and Ferenczi's aim were identical: to understand the functioning of telepathy and use this understanding in the analysis of the human psyche. Freud himself—who was much more cautious in this question than his innovative disciples, Jung and Ferenczi—used his observations on the functioning of telepathy in order to reinforce psychoanalytic theory. In his early writings on the subject, he debunked apparent telepathic occurrences in the same way as psychoanalysis did with every kind of supernatural belief system, religion, and symptom (Freud, 1904). Later, he admitted that telepathic phenomena could exist in some way (Brabant et al., 1993; Jones, 1957). It is important to note that the question of telepathy was the only manifestation of the supernatural whose existence was accepted by Freud: the only exception that was seemingly opposed to the materialistic, rationalistic approach of psychoanalysis. However, Freud supposed that telepathy could have a physical basis and worked similarly to the functioning of the telephone or the telegraph (Freud, 1933). From this point of view, he disconnected the concept of telepathy from the supernatural and the spiritual and considered it as any other psychological or physical problem. In this way, he maintained the framework of psychoanalysis in which superstitious beliefs and all apparently supernatural phenomena were debunked by psychoanalytic, materialistic terms. It must be added that the abovementioned efforts of Freud could have been connected with the fear and the repression of his own superstitious beliefs (Jones, 1957; Roustang, 1983). Several sources underlie the fact that in his private life Freud was not so skeptical towards the so-called occult, and he himself was also characterized by some superstitious beliefs (Freud, 1919; Jones, 1957).

It is not accidental that the problem of telepathy became an attractive field of research for many psychoanalysts. Among the different subjects that psychical researchers were interested in, telepathy was the only one that proved to be really relevant for the psychoanalysts. The reason for that was the strong connection between telepathy and the psychoanalytical situation (see Forrester, 1990). Later, some psychoanalysts realized that telepathic processes were strongly connected with the healing relationship (Deutsch, 1926; Hollós, 1933; Servadio, 1956). They supposed that the increased sensitivity, which characterizes the therapeutic rapport, could be the source of telepathy or thought-transference. Furthermore, they suspected that the telepathic message functions similarly to any other manifestation of unconscious processes and contents; according to their own observations, telepathic messages reflected the subjects' preconscious or unconscious complexes and belonged to the realm of primary processes (Hollós, 1933). Thus, they declared telepathy as an important field of psychoanalytical investigation, similar to neurotic symptoms or dreams.

When Ferenczi started to investigate so-called spiritualistic phenomena, psychoanalysis was only a nascent theory. After some lay observations in the field of spiritualism, he started to conduct scientific experiments with a few promising mediums. The first step in Ferenczi's telepathy experiments was his investigation with Frau Seidler, the divinator from Berlin. Although Frau Seidler showed extraordinary talent in reading unopened letters, when Ferenczi tried to convince Freud of the significance of her gifts, he had to face the resistance of his master. Freud was truly unconvinced of her abilities. As a result of this, Ferenczi had to find new subjects for the experiments. The Hungarian somnambulist Frau Jelinek was his second subject, who was unfortunately also unable to make a reliable impression on Freud (Brabant et al., 1993).

Finally, Ferenczi made great discoveries with a homosexual, masochistic patient, who often referred to Ferenczi's hidden thoughts in his free associations. This case proved to be convincing for Freud too, who abandoned his skepticism as a result of Ferenczi's account:

> Your—carefully preserved—observations on your masochist seem to me finally to shatter the doubts about the existence of thought-transference. Now it is a matter of getting used to it in your thoughts and losing respect for its novelty, and also preserving the secret long enough in the maternal womb, but that is where the doubt ends.
>
> (Brabant et al., 1993, p. 211)

From this time on, Ferenczi started to broaden the circle of investigations; he made observations on several of his patients and even with his fiancée, Gizella. However, his most successful experiments were those that he conducted with his homosexual patient. It slowly became clear to him that the process of telepathy was strongly connected with the transference situation. In 1910, he told Freud of his discovery:

> Interesting news in the transference story. Imagine, I am a great soothsayer, that is to say, a reader of thoughts! I am reading my patients' thoughts (in my free associations). The future methodology of CA must make use of this ... This method will be suitable to catch the patient's most active complexes at work—It can be refined even more! When I come to Vienna, I will introduce myself as "court astrologer of the psychoanalysts."
>
> (Brabant et al., 1993, pp. 235–236)

Although Freud shared Ferenczi's enthusiasm, his constant cautions bore witness to his basic ambivalence towards the question of telepathy. In 1910, Freud asked Ferenczi not to publish his results till 1913:

> I see destiny approaching inexorably, and I note that it has designated you to bring to light mysticism and the like, and that it would be just as futile as it is hard-hearted to keep you from it. Still, I think we ought to

> venture to slow it down. I would like to request that you continue to research in secrecy for two full years and don't come out until 1913; then, certainly, in the *Jahrbuch*, openly and aboveboard. You know my practical reasons against it and my secret painful sensitivities.
>
> (Brabant et al., 1993, pp. 239–240)

Ferenczi was obedient to his master and waited patiently. However, he did not publish his results in 1913. He only gave a paper to the Viennese Psychoanalytic Society, in which he summarized his experiences on thought-transference. His presentation was based on his telepathy experiments with the mediums Mr. and Mrs. Roth (Nunberg & Federn, 1975), but his results remained questionable for the audience. As a result of his failures to convince skeptical others, especially Freud, the problem of telepathy became less articulated in his letters and writings.

The Interpretation of Thought-Transference

Ferenczi had many different ideas on the possible basis of telepathic processes, but unfortunately none of them was well-elaborated. Rather, they were flexible ideas and meaningful observations, which outlined the later trends of research in this field of psychoanalysis. The core of his interpretation was his theory of introjection and projection, the processes that underlie the development of inner and outer reality and the boundaries of the self (Ferenczi, 1909, 1932b; Thurschwell, 1999, 2001). On the basis of these ideas, in 1910, he concluded the following: Anxiety reinforces the productivity of sending telepathic messages, while the calm state of mind increases the capacity for receiving telepathic messages. Furthermore, the receiver reacts unconsciously to thought-transference and activates those unconscious complexes that are closer to the unconscious complexes of the sender. The summation of personal complexes and the tendency of projection create the transference phenomena, which, depending on the predominance of introjection or projection, incline the individual to receive or send telepathic messages: "the paranoid is inclined toward projection and complex emanation, the hysteric toward introjection and complex resonance" (Brabant et al., 1993, p. 277).

Ferenczi says much more about the supposed mechanisms of thought-transference in his last work, the *Clinical Diary* (1932b). Placing the healing process on a metaphysical level, he speaks about a nonverbal healing force of the libido, which is based on the mysterious interconnectedness of the healer's and the patient's unconscious. According to Ferenczi, it is possible to react or resonate to somebody else's unconscious complexes, feelings, or thoughts in an unconscious way, which remains on the level of primary processes. The mysterious coincidences and telepathic occurrences are the manifestations of these hidden and latent perceptions and reactions.

This interconnectedness proved to be an exceptionally useful notion in the interpretation of telepathy; later several psychoanalysts, such as István Hollós (1933), Mihály Bálint (1955), and Nándor Fodor[4] (1947; Carrington & Fodor, 1953), applied this idea in their psychoanalytically oriented theories of telepathy. Among these interpreters, the problem of telepathy became a real psychoanalytic problem that was also as significant as any other aspect of the therapeutic situation. Not only was the psychoanalytic meaning of psychical phenomena searched by them, but the special connection between psychoanalytic transference and telepathy. According to Hollós and Bálint, telepathic occurrences develop in strong transference situations, in which the patient's past experiences are confused with the present situation and with the perception of the analyst. In Ferenczi's view, transference and countertransference were based on introjective and projective processes, in which the inner and the outer psychological contents could be changed and confused. Based on the special sensitivity that characterizes transference situations, not only did the transference of attitudes and emotions become theoretically possible, but also the transference of thoughts.

According to another of Ferenczi's ideas, the increased sensitivity, which characterizes some mental illnesses, could also be the key to telepathic capacities. In 1932, he wrote the following:

> From the very beginning I was inclined to think, that the hallucinations of the insane, or at least a part of them, are not imaginings but real perceptions, stemming from the environment and from the psyches of other human beings, which are accessible for them—precisely because of their psychologically motivated hypersensitivity—whereas normal people, focusing only on immediate matters of direct concern to them, remain unaffected. What comes to mind in this connection is the so-called occult powers of certain people, and the close relationship and easy transition between the two states: paranoia and psychic superperformance.
>
> (p. 58)

Elsewhere, he connects this increased sensitivity to the state of "dissolution" of the infantile psyche; from his point of view, this form of the psyche is much closer to the cosmic universe than is the developed adult psyche. Therefore, the abilities of mediums and supernormal qualities in general can be traced back to the wisdom and knowledge of children (Ferenczi, 1932b). Later, he interprets mediumism in terms of certain increased olfactory capacities that serve as the psycho-physiological explanation of mediumistic phenomena. According to this:

> A great deal of what has been regarded up to now as occult, or as a metaphysical superperformance, would thus become explicable in psycho-physiological terms. A further and still bolder step would then lead to the

> performances of spiritualist mediums, who can sense a person's total emanations, as they continue vibrating somewhere in space, even across the limitless passage of ages. (As a dog might [sense] the footprints of its deceased master.) Spiritualist mediums therefore reconstruct, with the aid of their sense of smell, a person's past. They may, aided by their olfactory imagination, follow a person back into the most distant past, to all the places he stayed in the course of his life.
>
> (p. 88)

It seems that some of Ferenczi's ideas on the interpretation of telepathy and mediumistic phenomena were based on purely psychoanalytical terms, while others—especially those that emerged at the end of his life—referred to a sort of spiritual understanding of the human psyche, in which the boundaries of the self and the body are flexible and undefined. In both cases, the connection between his interest in telepathy and psychoanalysis is rather obvious: It is about the unknown, hidden, unconscious capacity of the psyche, which serves not only the demystification of seemingly supernatural phenomena, but also the verification of the psychoanalytic theory of the unconscious. In this context, the existence of the human capacity to transfer thoughts bears witness to the hidden forces of the psyche; these forces are different from normal perception and cognition, and they refer to a radically different quality. The verification of such a different quality leads necessarily to the psychoanalytic concept of the unconscious for Ferenczi. From this point of view, Ferenczi's ideas on telepathy are a typical manifestation of psychoanalytical thinking, according to which every apparently mysterious or supernatural phenomenon can be understood and illuminated by using the theory of the unconscious, which explains them. However, he attributes further characteristics to the psychoanalytic concept of the unconscious. In Ferenczi's interpretations on telepathy, the unconscious is not a fixed intrapsychical entity, but a dynamic factor that is able to transgress the boundaries of the personal psyche.

It is also clear that Ferenczi's experiences in the field of psychical research are rather sporadic, and his theories on the subject are obviously unelaborated. Despite the fact that he was open to the possibility of psychical occurrences, he was a psychoanalyst at heart, and his primary field of interest was the psychoanalytical understanding of the human psyche. On the other hand, a significant part of his ideas on the possible functioning of telepathy emerged in connection with his ideas on transference and countertransference. In this sense, his experiences with telepathy are important supplements of his innovations. They refer to the changing and flexible borders of the human psyche that were the center of transference phenomena, introjection, and projection in Ferenczi's thinking. Taking into account all these facts, it is not surprising that some experts consider Ferenczi's psychical researcher activities outstanding and especially significant.

Why Was Ferenczi "One of the Most Adventurous Speculative Researchers" of the SPR?

In 1933, John Rickman, the English psychoanalyst and psychical researcher, wrote an enthusiastic obituary of Ferenczi in the *Proceedings of the Society for Psychical Research*. The obituary is surprising, since Rickman claims that Ferenczi was "one of the most adventurous speculative researchers" (p. 124) of the Society for Psychical Research, whose death is an enormous loss to the Society. In the introduction to the obituary, Rickman sets Ferenczi's psychical researcher activity in a radically new light:

> For over 30 years he published (first in Hungarian, later in German and English) papers on the phenomena of mental energy expressing itself in physical forms, the expression of instinctual longings in alterations of physiological states. The factors which lead to the employment of unusual physical means of expression were on the whole of less interest to him than the mechanisms of such "conversions from psychical to somatic" spheres, so he stood midway between the group of workers whose main interest is the effect of anxiety and guilt in mental life (the present-day tendency in psychoanalysis) and those whose work lies more especially in the descriptive field of psychical research. (p. 124)

Rickman's claim that Ferenczi was primarily interested in the conversions from psychical to somatic spheres seems to verify the significance of Ferenczi as a psychical researcher. In "The Phenomena of Hysterical Materialization" (1919), Ferenczi expressed himself clearly on the matter. In this paper, he points to the identity of the materialization phenomena in hysteria and mediumism. Although he does not delve into the problem of mediumistic materialization phenomena, it is rather clear that he was well aware of the potential significance of his ideas for psychical researchers.

According to Rickman, Ferenczi's most important work in the field of psychical research was his article on the "Stages in the Development of the Sense of Reality" (1913):

> His most important contributions bearing on psychical research lay in his stimulating papers on "The Development of the Sense of Reality," in which he showed how the child's developing perception of the external world is a slow relinquishing of phantasies and again how these phantasies are based on the child's notion of himself. In line with these researches are his penetrating observations on the way in which the mind, to conceal from itself its own defenselessness in the presence of what is felt to be overwhelming and disruptive internal excitement, either attributes to the external world what really belongs within itself or attributes to itself what is really external. (Rickman, 1933, p. 124)

From Rickman's point of view, the most significant aspect of the article is Ferenczi's attempt to grasp the development of the sense of reality in the interconnectedness of inner and outer reality. According to this, the infantile psyche is the source of outer reality just as outer reality is the source of the infantile psyche, since in the chain of introjections and projections the difference between the inner and the outer, the self and the non-self, is lost. What the child projects from itself becomes the so-called outer reality later. Ferenczi illuminates this early process in his paper "Introjection and Transference" (1909):

> We may suppose that to the newborn child everything perceived by the senses appears unitary, so to speak monistic. Only later does he learn to distinguish from his ego the malicious things, forming an outer world, that do not obey his will. That would be the first projection process, the primordial projection, and the later paranoiac probably makes use of the path thus traced out, in order to expel still more of his ego into the outer world.
>
> (p. 48)

Not only the newborn child and the paranoiac are characterized by introjective or projective processes. To a certain degree, every human psyche is built upon introjective and projective processes that create the inner subjective and the outer objective reality (Ferenczi, 1909). Although this idea can fertilize some theoretical branches of psychical research, remaining in the psychoanalytic framework, Ferenczi does not intend to touch on the question of psychical phenomena, but to describe a purely psychological process. However, it is probable that the psychoanalytically committed Rickman identified the functioning of introjective and projective processes with parapsychological phenomena. Since Rickman knew Ferenczi very well—he was a patient and disciple of his—the misunderstanding of Ferenczi's works is rather improbable. By the concepts of introjection and projection Ferenczi created a potential bridge between psychoanalysis and psychical research; although this bridge was not strong enough to generate remarkable cooperation, for those psychical researchers who were committed to psychoanalysis, it proved to be significant.

It must be added that analyzing the magical phase of development, Ferenczi referred to the possibility of telepathy in one of the footnotes of his article on "Stages in the Development of the Sense of Reality" (1913): "The psychological explanation of 'magic' naturally does not exclude the possibility of this belief containing also the foreshadowing of physical facts (telepathy, etc.)" (p. 230). Although his words are not really illuminating concerning his views on the connection between the development of the sense of reality and telepathy, by his remark he connected his psychoanalytical interpretation to the realm of psychical research. This remark is a typical example of the interconnectedness of Ferenczi's views on telepathy and his innovations. Psychical phenomena were not the focus of his theories, but by referring to them, Ferenczi gave a supplementary meaning of his theories by which psychical phenomena could have been understood in a psychoanalytic framework.

"Ferenczi's Evil Genius"

It seems very likely that Ferenczi's famous patient Elizabeth Severn (RN) also played a fundamental role in the evolution of Ferenczi's ideas on telepathy. Severn, labelled by Freud "Ferenczi's evil genius" (Jones, 1957, p. 407), had been Ferenczi's patient and disciple for the last eight years of his life. Taking into account the content of Ferenczi's later works and Severn's works on psychology and psychoanalysis, it is rather clear that they influenced each other not only on a psychoanalytical and emotional, but also on a theoretical level. The theory of mutual analysis was the result of this cooperation.

It is also likely that Severn's spiritualistic, mystical approach, which characterized her all of her life (Fortune, 1993, 1996), influenced Ferenczi. Although Severn was genuinely interested in psychoanalysis, in her own psychoanalytical theories she broadened the limits of psychoanalysis (Severn, 1919, 1933). The center of Severn's thinking was a non-psychoanalytical concept of the self, which had very clear spiritualistic connotations. In her book *The Discovery of the Self* (1933), she identified the self as follows:

> [The self is] the living, governing principle in man, the soul or mind which animates and gives meaning to all that he is and does. It is not only the "little I," the mere surface manifestation with which we are all more or less familiar, but a vital and integrating principle consisting of various and dynamic forces, which in their entirety make up the individual or Ego. It is the "big I," which having its roots not only in us but in the Cosmos, gives us intimations from time to time of vast processes, high aims, and even immortality. This internal entity is the representative of our higher or spiritual destinies, and is what gives significance to our whole existence.
>
> (p. 8)

Despite the cosmic connotations of the self, Severn used psychoanalytic concepts for the description of the psyche: Thus, her theory became a mixture of mystical and psychoanalytic ideas. According to Severn, the real core of the personality is not instinctual life but the above-described cosmic self. She united the materialistic and idealistic interpretations of life for the purpose of a new psychological science. In this new psychological approach, the body and the soul were interconnected; furthermore, the unconscious controlled all the physiological processes of the body.

She also criticized the rigidity of the classical psychoanalytical technique; according to her, the whole framework of psychoanalysis was too mechanistic and asymmetric. In contrast, she emphasized the necessity of love; in her view, the psychoanalyst has to be a parent, a better parent than the original one, who failed to support his or her child in the past. She also rejected the obligatory neutrality of the psychoanalyst; instead of this, she considered empathic feedback and emotional support fundamental.

It is obvious that the emphasizing of love and an empathic maternal attitude in the psychoanalytic situation is the same idea that characterized Ferenczi in his last years (Ferenczi, 1928, 1932a, 1932b). Their critiques of psychoanalysis are identical. It is likely that their conceptions emerged during their mutual analysis; however, it is still not clear who was the real source of these innovative ideas.

Nevertheless, taking into account the non-materialistic approach that characterized Ferenczi's later works, it is likely that the spiritualistic ideas of Severn played an important role in her relationship with Ferenczi, who was rather open to Severn's mystical beliefs. According to her, clairvoyance, precognition, or telepathy serves as an obvious proof for the unconscious dimensions of the psyche. In her understanding, telepathy is nothing other than the natural ability of the unconscious, which must be known and practiced. Her ideas on the therapeutic significance of telepathy are also remarkable: In her opinion, the psychotherapist is able to intrude into the psyche of the patient and thus create an identity between himself or herself and the sufferer. Although Severn does not use the word "telepathy" for this kind of relationship, it is evident that her ideas concerning this special identity are based on the functioning of telepathic processes. In this state of "psychical transfusion," there is no distance between the patient and the therapist; therefore, they share the same knowledge (Severn, 1933).

Severn's efforts to unite metaphysics and psychoanalysis were not fruitless. Partly thanks to her, the psychical researcher Nándor Fodor turned to psychoanalysis and later became one of the most prominent representatives of psychoanalytically interpreted psychical research. Ferenczi's influence on her theories is undeniable; it is also likely that Severn's mystical–spiritualistic approach impressed Ferenczi. Their later theories are the result of this cooperation, in which the materialist background of psychoanalysis was replaced by a cosmic, mystical interpretation of the psyche.

Psychical Research in Psychoanalysis

Although Ferenczi's ideas on the functioning of telepathy were not developed theories, they were undoubtedly interconnected with his innovative ideas. His interpretations on telepathy illuminated a supplementary meaning of transference, introjection, and projection, in which he transgressed the boundaries of the classical theory of psychoanalysis and developed a more permeable concept of the human psyche. From this point of view, it was not accidental that Ferenczi devoted an article to spiritualism in the first years of his psychological career. His interest in spiritualistic phenomena referred to the problem of psychological reality that he later interpreted by psychoanalytic terms. In this way, his experiences and views on telepathy were integrated in his psychoanalytic theories. Although his ideas on telepathy were not elaborated, the analysis of his interpretations proves that the core of his views on telepathy was his innovative theory on the flexible borders of the human psyche, introjection, and projection. The problem of telepathy became the problem of inner subjective and outer objective reality in his view.

The influence of Ferenczi's interest in telepathy was not manifested in spiritualistic views or mystical beliefs, but in those technical considerations that manifested themselves in connection with his ideas on telepathy. Based on his views on the permeability and sensitivity of the human psyche, Ferenczi developed a more emotional, symmetrical, and intuitive technique, in which the possibility of telepathic processes was also accepted. Taking into account the theoretical interconnectedness of Ferenczi's theories of telepathy and psychoanalytical innovations, it can be pointed out that the idea of the permeability of the psyche, which proved to be fundamental in Ferenczi's ideas of telepathy, fertilized Ferenczi's thinking and served as a basis for his greatest innovations, such as his unique view of transference and countertransference. According to the latter, the psychoanalyst's reactions and emotions are not avoidable artifacts of the psychoanalytic situation, but valuable and useful elements that create a more symmetric position in therapy. In this position, the therapist is also unconsciously involved in the psychoanalytic situation. His or her thoughts and emotions are potentially shareable on a conscious or unconscious level. Not only was the theory of mutual analysis developed on this basis, but also the theory of unconscious, telepathic communication. Following the footsteps of Ferenczi, Mihály Bálint (1955) describes very clearly the psychoanalytic significance of telepathy in psychoanalysis:

> These dynamic relations between transference and countertransference are, I think, important *contributory factors* in provoking apparently parapsychological phenomena during analytical treatment … If I am right, the crux of this involved relationship is the handling of the analyst's countertransference, especially the problem of how much and which side of this countertransference should be openly admitted, communicated, or "interpreted" to the patient.
>
> (p. 33)

According to Bálint—who developed his ideas following Hollós' (1933) theory on the telepathic occurrences in psychoanalysis—telepathic experiences occur in ambivalent and stressful analytic situations, when the analyst is unable to focus on the patient. However, because of technical reasons, the analyst decides to maintain the "façade of 'professional hypocrisy,' i.e., to pretend that all his interest and attention are still focused on the patient" (Bálint, 1955, p. 33). The patient's telepathic sensitivity is a reaction to the analyst's professional hypocrisy. It is easy to identify the influence of Ferenczi on Bálint's theory; the emphasis of countertransference, sensitivity, and the more symmetrical analytical situation refers to the innovative thoughts of Ferenczi.

It is not by accident that Ferenczi's fragmented ideas influenced so many psychoanalysts later. István Hollós (1933) developed his theory of telepathic occurrences between the patient and the analyst on the basis of Ferenczi's chance remark on the interconnectedness of the patient's and the analyst's unconscious. This idea and Hollós' theory proved to be significant in the works of Jule Eisenbud (1970), Emilio Servadio (1956, 1963), and Jan Ehrenwald (1947, 1954), who all tried to interpret the problem of telepathy and other psychical phenomena by using psychoanalytic theory. By doing so, they developed similar concepts on the flexibility and the sensitivity of the human psyche and the nature of the psychoanalytical situation as Ferenczi did. Nándor Fodor, the great Hungarian representative of psychical research and psychoanalysis, also knew Ferenczi and his theories, and partly as a result of his acquaintance with Elizabeth Severn, he developed a truly innovative way of psychoanalytical understanding of psychical phenomena (Fodor, 1934, 1959). His ideas on the parapsychological aspects of the psychoanalytic situation are much closer to the psychoanalysis of Ferenczi than to the psychoanalysis of Freud, which means that the integration of telepathy within psychoanalysis required very similar technical innovations that were present in Ferenczi. Taking into account the widespread effects of Ferenczi's fragmented theories, it cannot be accidental that John Rickman considers Ferenczi "one of the most adventurous speculative researchers" of the Society for Psychical Research. Not only did his articulated ideas influence the professional development of the abovementioned scholars, but the whole of Ferenczi's psychoanalysis, in which the flexibility of the boundaries of the psyche, its supposed permeability, the fundamental processes of introjection and projection, all refer to a great potential of psychical processes.

It is to be regretted that, in spite of the efforts of several psychical researchers and psychoanalysts (Carrington & Fodor, 1953; Mitchell, 1918, 1938), psychoanalytic ideas were not really applied in the field of psychical research. It is true that the rather complicated and often questioned scientific status of psychoanalysis made the desired cooperation with psychical research difficult. On the other hand, psychoanalysts also found it risky to undertake any significant connection or collaboration with the representatives of psychical research. Taking into account that several critiques of psychoanalysis tried to identify Freud's system with a sort of occult system, psychoanalysis had to distance itself from every kind of philosophy and practice that could have been connected with the so-called occult. In the eyes of Freud and his followers, psychical research had strong connections with those occult and spiritualist practices and philosophies, which they tried to demarcate from their own system (Jones, 1957). However, it is rather obvious that psychoanalysis was never as far from the "black tide of mud" of occultism (Jung, 1961, p. 173) as some representatives of it, especially Ernest Jones, wanted it to be. Ferenczi's works bear witness to this latent interconnectedness. Thus, Ferenczi's thoughts on telepathy illuminate both the relevance of psychical research to psychoanalysis and the relevance of psychoanalysis to psychical research.

Notes

1 This chapter originally appeared as: Gyimesi, J. (2012). Sándor Ferenczi and the problem of telepathy. *History of the Human Sciences, 25*, 131–148. Reprinted with permission.
2 István Hollós, a leading Hungarian psychoanalyst, a contemporary and colleague of Freud and Ferenczi.
3 In Hungarian, the word "spiritism" refers both to spiritism and to spiritualism.
4 Nándor Fodor, a psychical researcher and a psychoanalyst, a research officer of the International Institute of Psychical Research between 1934 and 1938.

References

Bálint, M. (1955). Notes on parapsychology and parapsychological healing. *International Journal of Psychoanalysis*, 36, 31–35.

Brabant, E., Falzeder, E., & Giampieri-Deutsch, P. (Eds.). (1993). *The correspondence of Sigmund Freud and Sándor Ferenczi, Vol. 1: 1908–1914*. Harvard University Press.

Carrington, H., & Fodor, N. (1953). *The story of the poltergeist down the centuries*. Hutchinson House.

Deutsch, H. (1926). Occult processes occurring during psychoanalysis. *Imago*, 12, 418–433.

Devereux, G. (Ed.). (1953). *Psychoanalysis and the occult*. International Universities Press.

Ehrenwald, J. (1947). *Telepathy and medical psychology*. Allen & Unwin.

Ehrenwald, J. (1954). *New dimensions of deep analysis: A study of telepathy in interpersonal relationships*. Allen & Unwin.

Eisenbud, J. (1970). *Psi and psychoanalysis: Studies in the psychoanalysis of psi-conditioned behavior*. Grune & Stratton.

Elekes, M. (1926). Az okkultizmus alapjelenségei. *Korunk*, May.

Ferenczi, S. (1899). Spiritism. *The Psychoanalytic Review*, 50A, 139–144.

Ferenczi, S. (1900a). Somnambulismus und spiritismus: Leopold Löwenfeld könyvének ismertetése. *Gyógyászat*, 40, 730.

Ferenczi, S. (1900b). Tanulmányok a szellemtan köréből (spiritizmus): Wajdits Lajos könyvének ismertetése. *Gyógyászat*, 40, 426.

Ferenczi, S. (1909). Introjection and transference. In J. Dupont (Ed.), *First contributions to psychoanalysis* (pp. 35–53). Karnac.

Ferenczi, S. (1913). Stages in the development of the sense of reality. In J. Dupont (Ed.), *First contributions to psychoanalysis* (pp. 213–239). Karnac.

Ferenczi, S. (1917). Barátságom Schachter Miksával. *Gyógyászat*, 52, 26–27.

Ferenczi, S. (1919). The phenomena of hysterical materialization. In J. Rickman (Ed.), *Further contributions to the theory and technique of psychoanalysis* (pp. 89–104). Hogarth Press.

Ferenczi, S. (1928). The elasticity of psychoanalytic technique. In M. Bálint (Ed.), *Final contributions to the problems and method of psychoanalysis* (pp. 87–102). Brunner/Mazel.

Ferenczi, S. (1932a). The confusion of tongues between adults and children: The language of tenderness and passion. In M. Bálint (Ed.), *Final contributions to the problems and methods of Psychoanalysis* (pp. 156–167). Karnac.

Ferenczi, S. (1932b). *The clinical diary of Sándor Ferenczi*. Harvard University Press.

Flournoy, T. (1900). *Des Indes à la planète Mars: Étude sur un cas de somnambulisme avec glossolalia*. Librairie Félix Alcan.

Fodor, N. (1934). *These mysterious people*. Rider.

Fodor, N. (1947). Telepathy in analysis. *Psychiatric Quarterly*, 21, 171–189.

Fodor, N. (1959). *The haunted mind: A psychoanalyst looks at the supernatural*. Garrett.

Forrester, J. (1990). Psychoanalysis: Gossip, telepathy and/or science. In *The seductions of psychoanalysis: Freud, Lacan, and Derrida* (pp. 246–260). Cambridge University Press.

Fortune, C. (1993). The case of "RN": Sándor Ferenczi's radical experiment in psychoanalysis. In L. Aron & A. Harris (Eds.), *The legacy of Sándor Ferenczi* (pp. 100–121). The Analytic Press.

Fortune, C. (1996). Mutual analysis: A logical outcome of Sándor Ferenczi's experiments in psychoanalysis. In P. L. Rudnytsky, A. Bókay, & P. Giampieri-Deutsch (Eds.), *Ferenczi's turn in psychoanalysis* (pp. 170–189). New York University Press.

Freud, S. (1904). A premonitory dream fulfilled. In G. Devereux (Ed.), *Psychoanalysis and the occult* (pp. 49–51). International Universities Press.

Freud, S. (1912). A note on the unconscious in psychoanalysis. In J. Strachey (Ed. & Trans.), *The standard edition of the complete psychological works of Sigmund Freud* (Vol. 12, pp. 257–266). Hogarth Press.

Freud, S. (1919). The uncanny. In J. Strachey (Ed. & Trans.), *The standard edition of the complete psychological works of Sigmund Freud* (Vol. 17, pp. 219–252). Hogarth Press.

Freud, S. (1921). Psychoanalysis and telepathy. In G. Devereux (Ed.), *Psychoanalysis and the occult* (pp. 56–68). International Universities Press.

Freud, S. (1922). Dreams and telepathy. In G. Devereux (Ed.), *Psychoanalysis and the occult* (pp. 69–86). International Universities Press.

Freud, S. (1933). Dreams and occultism. In G. Devereux (Ed.), *Psychoanalysis and the occult* (pp. 91–109). International Universities Press.

Hinshelwood, R. D. (1995). Psychoanalysis in Britain: Points of cultural access, 1893–1918. *International Journal of Psychoanalysis*, 76, 135–151.

Hollós, I. (1933). Psychopathologie alltäglicher telepathischer Erscheinungen. *Imago*, 19, 529–546.

Jaffé, A. (1971). *From the life and work of C. G. Jung*. Hodder & Stoughton.

James, W. (1886). Report of the committee on mediumistic phenomena. In F. H. Buckhart, F. Bowers, & I. K. Skrupskelis (Eds.), *Essays in psychical research* (pp. 14–19). Harvard University Press.
Janet, P. (1930). *L'automatisme psychologique*. Librairie Félix Alcan.
Jones, E. (1931). *On the nightmare*. Hogarth Press.
Jones, E. (1957). *The life and the work of Sigmund Freud, Vol. 3: The last phase 1919–1939*. Basic Books.
Jung, C. G. (1896). The border zones of exact science. In *The collected works of C. G. Jung* (pp. 5–19). Routledge & Kegan Paul.
Jung, C. G. (1897). Some thoughts on psychology. In *The collected works of C. G. Jung* (pp. 23–47). Routledge & Kegan Paul.
Jung, C. G. (1902). On the psychology and pathology of so-called occult phenomena. In *Collected papers on analytical psychology* (pp. 1–93). Moffat.
Jung, C. G. (1933). *Modern man in search of a soul*. Routledge.
Jung, C. G. (1944). *On the nature of the psyche*. Ark Paperbacks.
Jung, C. G. (1961). *Memories, dreams, reflections*. Fontana.
Jung, C. G. (1977). *Psychoanalysis and the occult*. Princeton University Press.
Jung, C. G. (2009). *The red book: Liber novus*. W. W. Norton.
Keeley, J. P. (2001). Subliminal promptings: Psychoanalytic theory and the society for psychical research. *American Imago*, 58, 767–791.
Luckhurst, R. (2002). *The invention of telepathy, 1870–1901*. Oxford University Press.
Mitchell, T. W. (1918). Psychology of the unconscious and psychoanalysis. *Proceedings of the Society for Psychical Research*, 30, 134–173.
Mitchell, T. W. (1938). The contributions of psychical research to psychotherapeutics. *Proceedings of the Society for Psychical Research*, 45, 175–786.
Myers, F. W. H. (1903). *Human personality and its survival of bodily death*. Longmans, Green.
Nunberg, H., & Federn, E. (Eds.). (1975). *Minutes of the Vienna psychoanalytic society* (Vol. 4). International Universities Press.
Oppenheim, J. (1988). *The other world: Spiritualism and psychical research in England, 1850–1914*. Cambridge University Press.
Richet, C. R. (1923). *Thirty years of psychical research: Being a treatise on metapsychics*. W. Collins & Sons.
Rickman, J. (1933). Obituary: Sándor Ferenczi. *Proceedings of the Society for Psychical Research*, 33, 124–125.
Roustang, F. (1983). *Psychoanalysis never lets go*. Johns Hopkins University Press.
Servadio, E. (1956). Transference and thought-transference. *International Journal of Psychoanalysis*, 37, 392–395.
Servadio, E. (1963). *Unconscious and paranormal factors in healing and recovery*. Society for Psychical Research.
Severn, E. (1919). *The psychology of behavior*. Dodd, Mead.
Severn, E. (1933). *The discovery of the self: A study in psychological cure*. David McKay.
Szántó, H. (1927). Nagy titkok küszöbén. Az okkult jelenségek filozó fiai mérlegelése. *Korunk*, 2, 1–10, 103–112.
Szilágyi, G. (1923). Der junge Spiritist: Ein psychoanalytisches Lebensbild. *Internationale Zeitschrift für Psychoanalyse*, 3, 402–427.

Thurschwell, P. (1999). Ferenczi's dangerous proximities: Telepathy, psychosis and the real event. *Differences*, 11, 150–178.

Thurschwell, P. (2001). *Literature, technology and magical thinking, 1880–1920*. Cambridge University Press.

Treitel, C. (2004). *A science for the soul: Occultism and the genesis of the German modern*. Johns Hopkins University Press.

Zumstein-Preiswerk, S. (1975). *C. G. Jungs medium: Die Geschichte der Helly Preiswerk*. Kindler.

Chapter 7

The Too Often Ignored Principles that Freud Enunciated about Telepathy[1]

Richard Reichbart

Richard Reichbart, Ph.D., distills from the four papers that Freud wrote on telepathy seven principles that Freud articulated about how to consider telepathy in the psychoanalytic process, how to process it, and how to recognize it as unconscious communication in the transference. These principles have been largely ignored by the psychoanalytic establishment, which has tended to look the other way and to relegate them to the psychoanalytic dustbin, despite the fact that the principles are very evident from Freud articles. At the end of this chapter, Richard summarizes each of the four telepathy articles written by Freud.

* * * *

Here is Freud, who became an honorary member of the British Society for Psychical Research in 1911, writing to the British psychical researcher Hereward Carrington in July 1921:

> I am not one of those who from the outset disapprove of the study of so-called occult phenomena as unscientific, as unworthy or even as dangerous. If I were at the beginning of a scientific career instead of now at its end, I would perhaps choose no other field of work in spite of all difficulties.
>
> (Freud, 1957, p. 12)

And in 1932, here he is writing to the Italian psychoanalyst Eduardo Weiss: "I am prepared to believe that behind all occult phenomena lies something new and important: the fact of thought transference, i.e., the transferring of psychical processes through space to other people" (Jones, 1957, pp. 453–454).

Yes, Freud was ambivalent about considering psychic processes, or what is in the parapsychological literature now called "psi phenomenon" or just simply "psi."[2] He could not entertain the concept of precognition or precognitive dreams, for example, and psychokinesis was far beyond him, but he believed in telepathy and, despite his ambivalence, he enunciated principles about its appearance in clinical practice, principles which to this day are accurate and applicable and which are more often than not forgotten by the psychoanalytic community.

DOI: 10.4324/9781003611042-8

I have extracted these principles from the four psychoanalytic articles that Freud published dealing with telepathy, and I have stated them in an express manner not only because they are important, but because there often seems to be resistance among psychoanalysts toward acknowledging how explicit Freud was when it came to dealing with telepathy in psychoanalytic process. In an addendum, after I present the principles, I summarize the four articles from which the principles are extracted for the reader who desires more complete references.

Here are the principles.

Telepathy Is a Common Phenomenon

In his 1933 paper "Dreams and Occultism," Freud stated that "if telepathy is a real process, we may suspect that in spite of it being hard to demonstrate, it is a quite common phenomenon" (p. 55). There is no indication on Freud's part, nor in my opinion does the rather vast parapsychological data indicate, that telepathy need to be only a consequence of a personality that has experienced early developmental trauma or separation, although of course in some individuals, as Ofra Eshel has so beautifully indicated, this can be a determining factor. Freud believed it was an integral part of daily life for everyone.

The State of Sleep Facilitates Telepathy

Again, in his 1933 paper, Freud emphasizes that the state of sleep "seems particularly suited for receiving telepathic messages." In such cases," he continues, "one has what is called a telepathic dream" (p. 37).

Telepathic Data Can Be Transmitted to a Person's Unconscious and Can Be Transformed in the Same Way as a "Day Residue" Would Be Transformed in the Manifest Content of a Dream

This is Freud's brilliant and intuitive assertion upon accepting telepathy (incidentally, one which it would be excellent that parapsychologists in general recognize, not only for dreams, but for determining whether a telepathic connection has taken place in general). As he says in 1922, "A telepathic message will be treated as a portion of the material that goes to the formation of a dream, like any other external or internal stimulus …" (Freud, 1922, p. 207). The example he gives is a dream by a man in which his wife gives birth to twins whose features and hair resemble his and his wife's; he then observes his wife giving the breast to one of the infants. In fact, the man's wife was deceased. It was his daughter who prematurely gave birth unexpectedly to twins and at a distance from her father.

Of the substitution of wife for daughter in the manifest content of the dream, Freud observes "how the telepathic message with the help of a lurking repressed wish became remodelled into a wish fulfillment" (p. 207). Concludes Freud:

> One forms the conviction that the telepathic news has played the same part as any other portion of the day's residues and that it has been changed in the same way by the dream-work and made to serve its purpose.
>
> (p. 207)

The Analyst Can Share Telepathic Data of Which the Patient May Not Be Aware to Make an Interpretation

Here, I must quickly recount The Forsyth Case from Freud's 1933 paper. A London doctor named Dr. Forsyth had just arrived to see Freud in the hope of arranging treatment with him. Freud did not have time to see him but took his card and arranged to talk later in the hope that he would acquire an excellent new patient. Freud's next patient was a Herr P., whom Freud despaired of curing of his sexual difficulties and who was not a particularly good "psychoanalytic patient." As soon as Herr P. arrived, he proceeded to tell Freud that a pretty virginal girl with whom he had a flirtation liked to refer to him as "Mr. Foresight." At this point, impressed by the possible psi circumstances, Freud showed Herr P. the card of Dr. Forsyth. What should the analyst do when, unbeknownst to the patient, something in the analyst's life has been revealed through a telepathic or psi communication? In this case, Freud steps out of anonymity and reveals something in his life to his patient. This in fact is the dilemma that each of the presenters here have had to address. Let me continue with the Forsyth case by enunciating another one of Freud's principles.

One Motivation for a Patient Unconsciously Evoking Psi Is to Compete with Other Patients for the Analyst's Attention

As Freud says, it was as if Herr P. was saying to him: "I'm a Forsyth too; that's what the girl calls me." And then Freud poignantly adds:

> It is hard to mistake the mixture of jealous demand and melancholy self-depreciation which finds its expression in this remark. We shall not be going astray if we complete it in some such way as this: It's mortifying to me that your thoughts should be so intensely occupied with this new arrival. Do come back to me: after all I'm a Forsyth too.
>
> (p. 51)

This dynamic appears frequently in telepathy in analytic process: Patients seek the analyst's attention, and of course this results in unconscious competition with other patients.

Eisenbud (1970) provides numerous examples of this. For example, a patient of mine, whose life was devoid of sexual intimacy, dreamt of being surrounded by numerous naked women from the exact same unusual vacation destination that another patient of mine had just visited with frequent sexual dalliances, as if to say to me: "I too am manly and desirable in this way. Look at me in my dream."

A Telepathic Episode Is Often a Function Not Only of Repression of Emotionally Charged Material by the Patient, but of Repression of Similar or Related Emotionally Charged Material of the Analyst

Freud did not specifically articulate this, but I contend the Forsyth case is actually of this nature, although Freud failed to realize this fact. But subsequent analysts have over and over recognized and commented about this, not just about traumatic events in the analyst's life that the patient telepathically picks up on—accidents, deaths, funerals (as in Ofra's example in Chapter 1) and medical issues (as in Janine's example in Chapter 3)—but also as I mentioned in Chapter 2 the analyst's embarrassing situations, such as not having enough cutlery for a dinner party (Pederson-Krag, 1953), a desire to wear a loud sports jacket (Eisenbud, 1946), or taking a chromium soap dish mistakenly shipped to him in a "spirit of belligerent dishonesty inspired by rising costs of his house undergoing renovation" (Ullman, 1973, pp. 50–51). In the Forsyth case, I argue that Freud himself contributed to the telepathy, because the Englishman Dr. Forsyth came to him through the intervention of Ernest Jones (who actually had by mistake interrupted a previous session with Herr P.), and Freud was at that time reading *The Forsyte Saga*, an English book that Jones favored. Jones was adamantly opposed to Freud's interest in telepathy, which Freud attributed at one point to Jones' overly sensitive "English sensibilities." So, it is as if Freud unconsciously was saying through the telepathic example: "I will show you, Jones: I will answer your sometimes insufferable fear mongering and skepticism about introducing psi into psychoanalysis by producing an example in which you yourself play a part. That will turn the tables so to speak and make my point."

When Psi Does Occur, Popular Explanations for Its Occurrence Need Not Be Accepted, and Other Hypotheses for Its Acceptance May Be More Accurate

Freud in effect announced this principle when he investigated the premonitions of psychics. A fortune teller predicted the crayfish poisoning of a brother-in-law of the patient who consulted her. However, the prophecy did not come true. But in fact, unbeknownst to the fortune teller, the brother-in-law had previously experienced crayfish poisoning. Freud hypothesized that his patient had aggressive wishes toward his brother-in-law that he be poisoned again, which the fortune teller telepathically received but attributed to the future. This principle is very important, one with which parapsychologists are very familiar but which at times Freud himself ignored. For example, if an apparition makes a seeming telepathic connection with a patient, it does not necessarily mean that the popular conceptions of apparitions have to be endorsed for the telepathy to have taken place … and conceivably with causal explanations that fall short of ghosts being the souls of dead people. For example, as I indicate in my book, one need not assume that the veridical information that the ghost of Hamlet's father conveys to Hamlet—that the father was poisoned—confirms that the ghost is the soul of the father. After all, the voluminous 1886 publication *Phantasms of the Living* by Gurney, Podmore, and Myers of the British Society for Psychical Research, involved a survey of 700 ghosts—of living persons—and contended that telepathy explained the phenomena.

These are seven of the principles that Freud formulated about how to think about and process telepathic events that occur in treatment. I have articulated them so didactically because they have been so often overlooked by those who are disinclined to recognize Freud's achievements in this area and who feel compelled to minimize or ignore them, often focusing on his ambivalence about telepathy rather than the principles he created despite his ambivalence.

The four telepathy articles from which Freud's principles are extracted are summarized here.

"Psychoanalysis and Telepathy" (1921)

This is Freud's first publication in which he discusses two prophecies of fortune tellers, and which also suggests one of the important principles. Freud comments on a fortune teller's prophecy concerning crayfish poisoning of the brother-in-law of a patient who sat for the fortune teller. The prophecy did not come true, but in fact the brother-in-law, unbeknownst to the fortune teller, had previously experienced crayfish poisoning. Freud hypothesizes that his patient had aggressive wishes toward his brother-in-law that he be poisoned again, which the fortune teller telepathically received but attributed to the future. The principle in effect is that telepathic messages can be shared, but that one can make false assumptions about their meaning; the popular way in which they are understood can be wrong, but that does not deny the fact that they may be examples of psi. A second example, also announcing the same principle, again suggests that a prophecy of a fortune teller was actually a product of telepathy rather than precognition. Years ago, the patient had consulted a fortune teller who, in predicting the future of the patient, apparently picked up telepathically on the history of the mother of the patient. The patient wished to have a life similar to her mother's, particularly to have two children before she was thirty—and in many respects subsequently did (thus the appearance of precognition by the fortune teller)—but according to Freud, what the fortune teller was in touch with *telepathically* was the patient's wish to be like the mother. Ehrenwald (2010), and then Brottman (2011), in a wonderful observation, state that the seemingly prophesying Witches of Thane in *Macbeth* might equally be considered to have telepathically picked up on Macbeth's desire to be king, and thus this too fits into Freud's examples.

"Dreams and Telepathy" (1922)

This second article of Freud's announces two important principles with regard to a possible telepathic dream that a father has concerning the birth of his daughter's twins that occurs at a distance from him. The initial principle announced is that the sleeping or dream state facilitates psi. The second, and a very important one, is that a telepathic message, unconsciously received, can be transformed in the manifest content of a dream in the same way that a day residue sensorily experienced is transformed.

Freud also makes some personal observations. He states of himself, "I have never had a telepathic dream" (p. 197). In addition, it should be noted that the twin-birth dream is not from his own practice; it is recounted in a letter from the dreamer. For the fact is, Freud observes that during "twenty-seven years of work as an analyst I have never been in a position to observe a truly telepathic dream in any of my patients" (p. 199). (This applies to telepathy in dreams, a statement he never contradicted later; but clearly he recounts an incident of putative telepathy in an analytic session with his patient Herr P. in the Forsyth case unrelated to a dream state.)

"The Occult Significance of Dreams" (1925)

This very short article repeats the fortune teller's prediction about the woman who subsequently had two children before she reached thirty (as her mother did), stressing the Oedipal dynamics of the wish because the patient was close to her father. In addition, Freud articulates the principle that telepathy is likely a common phenomenon, not necessarily dependent on early trauma of the person who communicates in this manner. Freud states this by speaking much more openly and positively about his own telepathic experiences and suggests that telepathic "transfer" is not unusual. He says:

> I have often had an impression, in the course of experiments in my private circle, that strongly emotionally coloured recollections can be successfully transferred without much difficulty. If one has the courage to subject to an analytic examination the associations of the person to whom the thoughts are supposed to be transferred, correspondences often come to light which would otherwise have remained undiscovered. On the basis of a number of experiences I am inclined to draw the conclusion that thought-transferences of this kind comes about particularly easily at the moment an idea emerges from the unconscious, or in theoretical terms, as it passes from the "primary process" to the "secondary process."
>
> (p. 138)

"Dreams and Occultism" (1933)

This posthumously published article is perhaps the most significant of the four Freud published. It contains the Forsyth case, the only reported case of Freud's involving telepathic material that took place during a patient's session with Freud. This was a case of telepathy in vivo, so to speak, in which Freud immediately mentioned to the patient, Herr P., the telepathy that had just occurred and analyzed the reasons for the telepathy with him. Of this example, Freud says it was "the one which left the strongest impression on me" (p. 47). Revealingly, the Forsyth case was supposed to be included in the earliest 1921 article, but because of what Freud recalls as his own "resistance," he mislaid his write-up of the case at the time and only found it later. Derrida (1988), in a brilliant discussion, makes much of this slip by Freud, which he also attributes to resistance, characterizing it as a "dis-association" and wondering whether psychoanalysis "must remain silent about the structure and the incorporation" of the "foreign body" of telepathy (p. 33). Ironically, then Derrida himself left out this material on telepathy from the book in which it was supposed to be published, requiring it to be published separately later!

In effect, three principles were expounded in this case. The first was that patients can invoke telepathy as a result of unconscious competitive feelings toward other patients, using telepathy to observe some aspect of the other patient's life and to gain the analyst's attention in preference to the other patient. The second and related principle is that patients can invoke telepathy by touching on the analyst's own life with similar motivations. The third principle, which has been expanded on by subsequent analysts, is that the analyst can break the analytic frame and inform the patient of the events or dreams he has telepathically (and unconsciously) picked up from the analyst's or another patient's life. By breaking the frame in this way, the analyst provides the patient with additional dynamic access to psi-mediated associations, dreams, or productions of which he would not otherwise have been aware.

In a broader sense, Freud states an overarching principle, citing a prior 1926 paper by Helene Deutsch (1953): It is that telepathy can be determined by the transference relations between patient and analyst.

Notes

1 This chapter is adapted from portions of "Psi and Psychoanalysis I: Rescuing Sisyphus" in *The Paranormal Surrounds Us: Psychic Phenomena in Literature, Culture and Psychoanalysis* (Reichbart, 2019).

2 The use of the term and symbol "psi" (the 23rd letter of the Greek alphabet) to represent psychic phenomena was introduced by the psychologist Robert Thouless in a 1942 *British Journal of Psychology* article, three years after Freud's death (Willin, 2021).

References

Brottman, M. (2011). *Phantoms of the clinic: From thought transference to projective identification*. Karnac.

Derrida, J. (1988) Telepathy (N. Royal, Trans.). *Oxford Literature Review*, 10 (3), 3–41.

Deutsch, H. (1953). Occult processes occurring during psychoanalysis. In G. Devereux (Ed.), *Psychoanalysis and the occult* (pp. 133–146). International Universities Press.

Ehrenwald, J. (2010). An autobiographical fragment. In R. Pilkington (Ed.), *Esprit: Men and women of parapsychology* (pp. 36–44). Anomalist Books.

Eisenbud, J. (1946). Telepathy and problems of psychoanalysis. *Psychoanalytic Quarterly*, 14, 32–87.

Eisenbud, J. (1970). *Psi and psychoanalysis: Studies in the psychoanalysis of psi-conditioned behavior*. Grune & Stratton.

Freud, S. (1921). Psychoanalysis and telepathy. In J. Strachey (Ed. & Trans.), *The standard edition of the complete psychological works of Sigmund Freud* (Vol. 18, pp. 177–193). Hogarth Press.

Freud, S. (1922). Dreams and telepathy. In J. Strachey (Ed. & Trans.), *The standard edition of the complete psychological works of Sigmund Freud* (Vol. 18, pp. 197–220). Hogarth Press.

Freud, S. (1925). The occult significance of dreams. In J. Strachey (Ed. & Trans.), *The standard edition of the complete psychological works of Sigmund Freud* (Vol. 19, pp. 125–138). Hogarth Press.

Freud, S. (1933). Dreams and occultism. In G. Devereux (Ed.), *Psychoanalysis and the occult* (pp. 91–109). International Universities Press.

Freud, S. (1957). An unpublished letter on parapsychology. In N. Fodor (Trans.), *Psychoanalysis and the future* (pp. 12–13). National Psychological Association for Psychoanalysis.

Gurney, E., Myers, F. W. H., & Podmore, F. (1886). *Phantasms of the living* (Vol. 1). The Society for Psychical Research.

Jones, E. (1957). *The life and the work of Sigmund Freud, Vol. 3: The last phase 1919–1939*. Basic Books.

Pederson-Krag, G. (1953). Telepathy and repression. In G. Devereux (ed.), *Psychoanalysis and the occult* (pp. 277–287). International Universities Press.

Reichbart, R. (2019). *The paranormal surrounds us: Psychic phenomena in literature, culture, and psychoanalysis*. McFarland.

Ullman, M. (1973). Dream telepathy: Experimental and clinical findings. In N. Totton (Ed.), *Psychoanalysis and the paranormal: Lands of darkness* (pp. 15–46). Karnac.

Willin, M. (2021). Robert Thouless. In *Psi encyclopedia*. The Society for Psychical Research. Retrieved from https://psi-encyclopedia.spr.ac.uk/articles/robert-thouless.

Chapter 8

Telepathy—An Expanded Perspective

Implications for Clinical Practice and Beyond

Ruth Rosenbaum

In this chapter, Ruth Rosenbaum, Ph.D., from the National Psychological Association for Psychoanalysis (NPAP) in New York City, suggests the need for an expanded conceptualization of the unconscious, which she describes as a "nonlocal unconscious," in order to accommodate the implications of telepathy that challenge our usual assumptions about time, space and the very nature of our reality. She presents clinical material, including an emotionally moving case that involved the collapse of the twin towers in New York City on September 11, 2001, to illustrate a continuum of types of telepathic activity in psychodynamic practice. Her discussion integrates concepts like mirror neurons, nonlocality and entanglement suggesting that telepathy reflects a fundamental interconnectedness of human existence. Thus, drawing from neuroscience and quantum physics, she shows the potential for the psychoanalytic encounter with telepathy to become an important part of an interdisciplinary exploration.

* * * *

Introduction

This chapter begins at a place of acceptance of telepathy as a verifiable phenomenon, as demonstrated in several contributions to this book, and explores the questions it raises. In 1933, Freud wrote: "If one gets used to the idea of telepathy one can account for a great deal by means of it" (p. 108). But what accounts for telepathy? Specifically, what is the elusive medium via which the often stunning telepathic transfer of information occurs, and what are its implications for psychoanalytic theory and practice and for understanding the nature of the reality that underlies our existence? In pursuing answers to these questions, the author points to an implicit conversation emerging between psychoanalysis and several of the "hard sciences" that are openly grappling with many of the same questions posed to us by instances of telepathy. They are encountering a similar "slipperiness" of empirical evidence for their theories that has long been the basis of scientific critique of psychoanalytic theory and practice.

DOI: 10.4324/9781003611042-9

Given the shift in perspective on the boundaries between self and other, and a rethinking of notions of time and space that a serious consideration of telepathy demands, the author proposes the need for a re-visioning of the unconscious. Expanding beyond the framework of contemporary theories of the dyadic expansion of consciousness, the relational unconscious, and the intersubjective "indissoluble psychological system" (Atwood & Stolorow, 1984, p. 64) co-created by patient and therapist, the author proposes the concept of "the nonlocal unconscious." Just as Freud moved from the topographic model to the dynamic model of fluctuating relationships between id, ego, and superego as he discovered more about unconscious processes, we need to consider a yet more comprehensive conceptualization of the unconscious in light of growing acknowledgment in our field and others of forms of communication, telepathy being one of them, that defy the paradigm to which we are accustomed regarding how communication takes place.

The cases presented in this chapter reflect a continuum of different kinds of telepathic communication, each illustrating a different "dialect" of the language by which the nonlocal unconscious communicates. In the main case presented, the author illustrates how awareness of telepathy as a derivative of a fundamental nonlocal unconscious points toward a different kind of attention regarding countertransference analysis and therapeutic action, particularly in instances of stuck-ness or impasse in psychotherapy.

Passion at a Distance

An interesting irony has emerged in the last 20 years: There has been an accumulation of studies (Abbass et al., 2006; Driessen et al., 2013; Huber et al., 2012; Leichsenring & Klein, 2014; Leichsenring et al., 2014; Shedler, 2010, 2016; Turner et al., 2008; Yakeley, 2014) demonstrating empirical evidence for the efficacy of psychoanalytic therapies, showing greater effect size and longer duration of positive outcome for a wide array of serious mental health problems than in many other therapies, allowing us, finally, a seat at the adult's table of empiricism. Yet, at the same time, several of the hard sciences, known for insisting on rigorous standards of empirical evidence, have been speaking a language of poetic speculation and empirical uncertainty, not unlike that which emerges from the complexity of analytic treatment and interpretation.

In fact, many scientists, in an attempt to understand a dimension of our reality that is beyond the realm of empiricism, resonate with Bion's (1970) concept of "O," an infinite, unknown, and unknowable dimension of our existence, unreachable through knowledge, and with Lacan's (1991) idea of the Real, which he states "is what resists symbolization absolutely" (p. 66).

Recently, some major players in the fields of cosmology and quantum physics have suggested that they set aside the need for experimental confirmation of even the most respected and enduring theories about our universe. They acknowledge that their theories are not able to fully account for the existence of our universe.

(Even the Big Bang and string theories rest on shaky evidential ground.) As one critic said, "They are breaking with centuries of philosophical tradition of defining scientific knowledge as empirical" (Ellis & Silk, 2014, p. 321). However, in both science and psychology, theories are ever-evolving approximations of aspects of our existence that may never amount to definitive proofs that stand the test of time. Freud would agree: "It is a mistake," he said, "to believe that a science consists of nothing but conclusively proved theorems, and any such demand would be unjust" (Freud, 1920, p. 33). It is interesting that he made this statement in 1920, at the dawn of the official emergence of the theory of quantum mechanics, which supplanted, after two and half centuries, the reign of Newtonian physics by presenting a more complex and comprehensive depiction of the foundations of our reality, one which abounds in uncertainty. Several highly respected physicists have spoken openly of the acceptance and integration of telepathy and other anomalous forms of communication into the framework of scientific theory, particularly quantum mechanics. Among them, Henry Margenau, Yale University physicist and member of Princeton University's Institute for Advanced Study, stated:

> Strangely, it does not seem possible to find the scientific laws or principles violated by the existence of (these phenomena). We can find contradictions between their occurrence and our culturally accepted view of reality—but not—as many of us have believed—between their occurrence and the scientific laws that have been so laboriously developed.
>
> (LeShan, 1987, p. 119)

Another physicist, O. Costas de Beauregard (1998), wrote that the concept of "nonlocality" in "today's physics requires the possibility … of the existence of so-called 'paranormal' phenomena such as telepathy, precognition and psychokinesis" (p. 315).

Locality in physics refers to the realm of linear measures of time and space, and of actions and predictable reactions, as described by Newtonian physics. The concept of nonlocality rests on an impenetrable oxymoron—it refers to a space without location, a dimensionless dimension, with no resemblance to the measurable grid of time and space on which our daily lives depend. This "space" is always present, albeit intangible, within reach of our unconscious, and at times moving into our conscious awareness and experience. I say it is always present because, just as dreams exist whether or not we remember them, and whether or not they offer themselves to our conscious mind for interpretation, telepathic communication is a fundamental property of our minds, even if it doesn't always rise to the level of conscious awareness or present itself to us in ways that can be easily tracked or proven.

Discoverers of mirror neurons explain that we all participate in a "shared intersubjective space" (Gallese, 2003, p. 160), characterized by an "unmediated resonance" (Goldman & Sripada, 2005, p. 207), "unmediated" pointing to a profound pre-existing interconnectedness. (To clarify mirror neuron activity: If I raise my hand, the very same neurons in my brain that enable me to do that are automatically fired in your brain as you observe me raising my hand.) We think of empathy as putting ourselves in another's shoes, but mirror neuron activity suggests that we are also automatically, without conscious effort, in each other's shoes. One of the mirror neuron researchers whom I interviewed suggested that our brains may be wired for access to a domain beyond the physical domain in which the wires (or neurons) themselves exist. In other words, our brain, in addition to all its essential functions, may serve as a portal to a nonmaterial domain that exceeds its own material existence. Off the record, he told me that he thinks that mirror neurons may one day account for telepathy. (When he said this, he had no idea of my interest in the topic, at least not consciously.)

Often, the concept of entanglement from quantum physics is summoned in attempts to understand telepathy. However, most physicists caution that the two can be related only as a poetic analogy or metaphor. Entanglement describes the phenomenon when two photons (light particles) separated at a source traveling great distances from each other (as in experiments of up to 12,000 miles of separation) instantaneously coordinate aspects of spin and charge, seeming to "know" each other's characteristics without any signal or known form of energy passing between them. When we consider that our brains contain 86 billion neurons, amounting to an estimated 100 trillion synaptic interconnections, with each neuron containing roughly one quadrillion atoms (each of which consists of innumerable subatomic particles), this staggering complexity does not allow for a direct comparison to the entanglement of two photons. However, what we can say is that in the case of both entangled photons and the intermingled mental experiences involved in telepathy, each points to a communication of information that defies empirically traceable modes of information transfer. Einstein referred to the photons' inscrutable behavior as "spooky action at a distance" (Lindley, 1996, p. 8). However, as physicist Abner Shimony commented, the word "action" is not applicable, because no signal could be involved in the photons' simultaneous coordination of spin and momentum. He thus coined the rather poetic phrase "passion at a distance" (Howard, 2009, p. 3). (He may not have had this in mind, but "passion at a distance" mirrors the Greek roots of the word telepathy: *tele* meaning distant, and *pathos* meaning intense feeling, passion.) In fact, Shimony thought of the entangled photons as "feeling one another's presence and properties enough to ensure the strong correlations" (p. 3) in their properties.

I have taken the liberty of borrowing Shimony's phrase "passion at a distance" to epitomize the therapeutic relationship, wherein two seemingly separate minds participate in a uniquely intimate space with an emotional intensity and passion that facilitates the blurring of personal boundaries, and the feeling of "one another's presence and properties."

It is important to note that though intimate bonds, such as patient and therapist, close friends, lovers, and twins, seem to facilitate the experience of telepathy, the nonlocal interconnectedness suggested by telepathy extends to situations involving total strangers. If, as I suggest, the telepathic continuum is a basic underpinning of our reality, it makes sense that it would not be limited in its potential effects to specific circumstances. For example, remote viewing experiments conducted by, among others, the Stanford Research Institute, funded by the CIA, the Defense Intelligence Agency, the Army, Navy, and NASA, demonstrated that subjects were able to draw or describe an undisclosed, randomly selected target site that was visited and observed by another person totally unknown to the subject. The accuracy rate of these remote viewings was four standard deviations from what would be expected by chance (Targ, 2019, p. 569). Another form of nonlocal unconscious communication, called influencing at a distance, has been highlighted in several studies in peer-reviewed journals, showing strong evidence that one person or a group of people can influence at a distance the mental state, physiological measures, even rates and specific measures of healing after cardiac surgery, of another person or people who are unaware of the intention in question (Braud & Schlitz, 1991; Byrd, 1988; Harris et al., 1999; Schmidt, 2012). These studies demonstrate that conscious intention may sometimes play a facilitative role in initiating distant effects, suggesting that our conscious minds have the potential to activate and influence nonlocal unconscious communications between people, unmediated by any discernible signal, yet producing measurable effects.

Some scientists suggest that the human unconscious shares an interface or "pre-distinction continuum" with the intangible domain described by quantum physics, characterized by nonlocality, and that the interface may be a portal for the emergence of derivatives such as telepathy, influence at a distance, and other psi phenomena (Jahn & Dunne, 2001). Similarly, Jung (1952) also theorized that the unconscious could engage in "a space–time continuum where space is not space, and time not time" (p. 75), and carry knowledge from it into conscious awareness.[1]

Our observations and perceptions are informed far more by our unconscious than our conscious minds. It is thought by many neuroscientists that 95% of our experience is determined by our unconscious. On the level of sensory perception alone—of what we perceive through our material, local, sensory systems—it has been estimated that we receive and process 11 million bits of information every second, of which only between 16 and 40 bits reach conscious awareness (Norretranders, 1998, pp. 125–126). Imagine, then, the exponential information-gathering capacity of the nonlocal, extrasensory aspect of our unconscious, and the potential variety of ways in which information from a quantum field with boundless possibilities can be conveyed to our conscious minds.

Adjusting the Lens

To preface the first case I'll describe: We know from quantum physics that every observation affects the observed, and in the context of psychoanalytic intersubjectivity theory, the observed is also observing and affecting the observer, creating an ongoing Moebius strip of mutual influence and shaping on both conscious and unconscious levels. Each one of us observes with a different set of lenses depending on theory, past experience, personal beliefs, and defenses. Because of the unusual responsibility entrusted to us as therapists, we need to continually examine our filters and refine ourselves as observers, depending on the particular patient and on what is happening in the treatment. If we keep in mind that telepathy is a derivative, a precipitate, of a nonmaterial domain accessible to our nonlocal unconscious, and an indication of the extent to which we are in each other's shoes, we might focus more attention on countertransference analysis as an active process of reshaping ourselves as instruments of observation. I have found this perspective especially helpful in instances of stuck-ness or impasse in therapy, as I hope to illustrate in the case of Mike.

Mike, a man in his late thirties, who worked as a paralegal in a large firm, came to see me in early 2002. He entered my office in a whoosh of agitated energy, and sitting down with an emphatic sigh, he began: "I really need help, but I can't get it! I haven't slept in months, and all I wanted was something to help me sleep. Two psychiatrists told me I was schizophrenic, and they both said they couldn't give me sleep medication until I took other medications for the schizophrenia to see how I adjusted to them. So I tried some of the medication, but I stopped a few weeks ago—it was making me crazy!"

I soon learned that on September 11, 2001, Mike was in his office in one of the buildings near the World Trade Center when the planes hit the towers. He made his way home, one of the hundreds of ghoulish figures walking over the Brooklyn Bridge, covered in the ash and particles of buildings and bodies. Puzzled, as I saw his symptoms in keeping with what I had seen in other 9/11 survivors, I asked him how he'd understood the diagnoses of schizophrenia. "I just told them the truth," he said, watching me cautiously, waiting for my response as he explained: Starting shortly after 9/11, on most nights, he told me that he was visited by several of the deceased souls who'd died in the moments when the planes hit the Towers. "They were really lost souls," he said sadly. "Some of them didn't even know they were dead. I think they were drawn to me so I could help them move on, you know, go to the light. But they just won't go! And I can't sleep!" It seemed that these souls were besieging him with their anguish and confusion, and a few were obsessed with unfinished business. One woman, he recounted, from Cantor Fitzgerald (the company that suffered the greatest losses), was distressed because she hadn't completed work on a big account and kept pleading with Mike to make an important call for her that had been abruptly interrupted by the attack. And a man who had brought a special gift for his fiancé to the office that day, planning to give it to her when they met for dinner that night—a night that never came—asked Mike to find the gift and get it to her.

As time went on, I learned that Mike thought of himself as a healer and so, felt a responsibility to help. At first, he gently tried to get them to realize they were dead and help them "move on." But, sleep-deprived and experiencing his own PTSD, he became impatient and would adopt an arrogant, bossy attitude, often peppering his speech with four-letter words. In his day-life, too, though he spoke of wanting to help people, his relationships both at work and in his personal life were often filled with conflict, with Mike's anger and frustration taking center stage, not unlike the way he related to some of the deceased visitors. This pattern had been in place well before 9/11, resulting in some clashes at work with both his boss and co-workers, at times threatening his employment. He also had on-and-off feuds even with close friends, with long periods of estrangement. As we explored the dynamics and defenses that had developed in childhood that contributed to this pattern, I decided to focus on his interactions with both the deceased and the living, since the patterns that emerged with both were very similar.

Mike's childhood was one of emotional chaos. He was painfully shy, and his hardworking parents were ill-equipped to deal with the anxieties, fears and hopes of this bright, sensitive child. Subjected to cruel mocking and bullying by classmates, he often left school with bruises and bleeding from fights he had no chance of winning. The only safe harbor amid the violence and painful humiliation was Connie, his maternal grandmother. Connie lived just a few blocks away, and Mike would go to her house as much as possible, receiving salve for his cuts and bruises and unconditional love , as he listened to her stories about her childhood in Italy. Connie had a reputation for having deceased family members come to her in dreams, alerting her to when a living family member or friend was going to get sick or die; apparently, she was eerily accurate.

When Mike was 12, Connie and her husband moved to a different state. Mike was devastated. To make matters worse, he was to enter a new school that fall and wasn't prepared for the bullying and violence that went well beyond what he'd experienced in grade school. One day, in eleventh grade, as he was about to leave the school, Mike saw the school's head bully sauntering toward him down the hallway, shouting familiar taunts. Mike started to turn and run, his usual reflex, but as he recounted:

> Something snapped in me, I'd had it. I couldn't run anymore. I don't even think I knew what I was doing, I ran toward him, grabbed him with all my strength and shoved him so hard against the wall, he was bleeding. We both got suspended for three days, but I tell you, no one ever touched me again.

After that, verbal bullying became a way of being for him. It earned him the only sense of protection he'd ever felt outside of Connie's house, and it became his calling card. He had always been averse to physical violence, so after he "conquered" the school bully, he turned to words and an aggressive tone to show "muscle" right away, no matter the situation. We explored the extent to which this patterned permeated and limited his relationships.

I want to mention one more symptom that developed after 9/11. It was an extreme, rather sudden loss of all of his body hair. When I first met him, I assumed his black painted-on eyebrows were an intentional part of his theatrical presentation, but it turned out they were a necessary replacement. He'd gone to several doctors, but none of the tests revealed any change in his hormones or other blood markers. It was assumed to be a severe stress response to his 9/11 experience, but after the initial shock and accommodation to his "new body," it didn't seem to cause him much distress—in fact, I thought that he experienced it as a kind of "badge of courage," a somatic certification of his having both endured and survived the trauma of 9/11.

Sleep deprivation was an increasing threat to Mike's health and well-being, but he refused to go to yet another psychiatrist. After some time, I found a psychiatrist at one of the major New York hospitals who was from a South American culture. My hopeful hunch was that the lens through which he would see Mike's experience might be different enough to avoid another diagnosis of schizophrenia. Very reluctantly, Mike agreed to see him. When he came in for his session with me after seeing the psychiatrist, he smiled triumphantly and waved the prescriptions for anxiety and sleep he'd been given. He proceeded to tell me about the great conversation he had with the "doc." He told him about Connie's prescient dreams, and the psychiatrist told Mike that where he came from, it was not uncommon for people to receive messages from dead ancestors, and there were special shamanic figures who helped the deceased transition after death. It was clear that Mike saw himself as an American shamanic figure, albeit one now thwarted in his mission by the frustrating resistance to his efforts by the nightly visitors.

The anxiety and sleep medication helped; Mike was able to get some sleep, despite the ongoing presence of the restless souls in his bedroom at night. His efforts to understand and try to temper his bullying reactions when people in his life didn't follow his advice were beginning to bring about some changes. He even reached out to one of his friends from whom he'd been estranged. I wondered, then: Why was there not similar movement with respect to the deceased? They were still there most nights, and the conflict with some had even escalated. In one go-around with the Cantor Fitzgerald woman, he told me he'd yelled at her:

> WILL YOU STOP WITH YOUR FRIGGIN' PHONE CALL, MOVE ON, I TOLD YOU, YOU'RE DEAD!

It occurred to me that something was compelling him to hold on to them as much as they seemed to be holding on to him. It appeared as though he was stuck, along with them, in that moment of horror and shock when the planes hit the towers. His experience of their inability to "move on" was, at least in part, I thought, a displacement of his difficulty dealing with his own 9/11 trauma. But I also had to consider my potential contribution to the collective stuck-ness all of us were experiencing. I thought this might have been because Mike was missing something in our connection that he found in his connection to the deceased—perhaps the identification with Connie and her communing with long-gone ancestors made him feel a depth of security and connection that he didn't feel with me. Had I, unconsciously, become complacent, too comfortable with Mike's positive transference, his often-expressed appreciation of me as understanding, non-judgmental, and open to his experiences?

I had to go deeper to understand myself as an observational instrument. With some patients, being in the space with them might require, for deep healing of early empathic failures, a less boundaried kind of empathy and an intentional movement toward that unmediated, nonlinear resonance spoken about by the pioneers in neuroscience and quantum physics. There are, I believe, increments of states of oneness and degrees of empathy, and I needed to see more clearly where I was on that continuum. With no expectation of a particular outcome, I thought of a way to explore this, and, at very least, to get closer to Mike's experience.

Shortly after 9/11, I had received some referrals of first responders, firemen and policemen who worked at ground zero, digging in the fuming piles of debris and death. Two of them, both firemen from different companies, each told me of experiences they had early in the morning when they arrived at Ground Zero. As one said, "Ruth, you're going to think I'm crazy. But I have to tell you, I can't even tell my wife, and definitely not my priest ..." He paused, drew a big sigh, and said, "Some mornings, I'm down there before dawn, and I swear, I see these vapory figures, and I hear, I swear, I'm not hallucinating—I hear the most horrible moans and gasps; it takes my breath away. I know this sounds crazy, but I think it's the spirits of some of the people who died so suddenly, like they're just caught there, right in that horrible moment. Do you think I'm crazy?"

It was several weeks after I began to work with the firemen that I met Mike for the first time. As Mike struggled with the deceased, in thinking about myself as the observational instrument, I realized that I had taken in the firemen's accounts in a different way than I had Mike's. I metabolized their words without any impediment in my unconscious. Though I was empathic, present, and intrigued by Mike's ongoing interactions with the deceased, and very fond of him, I realized I'd only partially digested his experience. I had to acknowledge that firemen resided in my psyche as cultural icons, heroes, especially in the context of the sacrifices they made on 9/11. Because of this difference in deep, unconscious associations, I had not been the same observer for Mike as I had been for the firemen.

Hoping simply to adjust my lens to deepen my perspective on Mike's experience, and without any particular expectation, I arrived at the following plan: In the weeks after 9/11, most days the *New York Times* published a number of profiles with pictures of the people who had died on that day. I'd read most of them and saved some. I dug through the disorganized pile of papers I save to read or re-read and found them. Most nights after work I read several of them, absorbing myself in a kind of meditation, allowing myself to feel the fullness of the lives I imagined from the profiles and the searing pain as I imagined their sudden horrifying deaths.

One night, as I read through several profiles, I came across one of a woman who immediately brought to mind the Cantor Fitzgerald woman who was still so annoying to Mike. He'd spoken about her so much that a vague, visual impression of her had developed in my mind. The woman in the *Times* profile resembled my image somewhat. But it was the description of her that really drew my attention. She was described as a well-liked and respected super-employee with a great deal of responsibility, known for being extremely reliable, competent, and conscientious. It seemed she would be someone who would be very upset if she hadn't completed an important call for her boss. Following this discovery, though I continued reading some of the others, I would always go back to this woman's profile, allowing myself to experience her as the actual woman who was, out of her desperation and confusion, harassing (as he put it) Mike at night.

A few weeks after I first began to read the profiles, Mike came into his session very excited about a dream he'd had. He plopped down on the couch and began:

> "Connie visited me in a dream. It's about time! I don't know what took her so long, you know, with 9/11 and all! Anyway, she was wearing a yellow striped apron like the one she'd be wearing in the kitchen when I went to her house after school. In the dream she looked me right in the eye and told me she's a big fan of yours. She told me I'm in good hands—I'm safe."

After digesting the likelihood that he hadn't felt totally safe with me until this point, I thought that his dream, and the timing of it, indicated that Mike's unconscious "knew" about the changes that occurred in my own unconscious, changes that were a result of my conscious efforts to alter my mode of observing his experience. This process seemed to be a catalyst for a deeper sense of trust and safety.

And then, about three weeks later, something very unexpected occurred. There is a long hallway between my entrance door and my office room, and usually, as we would enter the office together, I would sit down in my chair, and Mike would walk over to the couch opposite me. But this time, he came right over to where I sat and leaned over, his face quite close to mine, pointing to the side of his face: "Take a look!" At first, I couldn't see anything; he leaned his face closer and pointed again—and then I saw it—barely perceptible, but definitely there: a thin layer of fuzz. His beard had begun to grow. Over the next month, his eyebrows began to grow back, and, he told me, all his body hair was coming back.

We reflected on this together: The last time he'd felt unconditional love, understanding, and protection was just before Connie moved and just before he'd entered puberty. I told him that for many people the trauma of 9/11 seemed to revive experiences of earlier trauma, including flashbacks and nightmares of long-ago traumatic events, and for some time the past and present traumas' effects blended together. After his experience on 9/11, it seemed that Mike's entire system had been in need of something to hold on to for a feeling of comfort and protection after the planes hit. In this case, his vulnerable system seemed to have found a way to re-create aspects of a pre-pubescent body, reminiscent of the state he was in before the shock of Connie's move and the subsequent escalation of violence toward him in high school. I thought of how similar that "holding on" was to the ways in which Mike's nightly visitors were clinging to their final pre-trauma moments, when life was safe and predictable. Once Connie appeared in his dream and gave me her official stamp of approval, he could "move on" psychologically and physically, on both conscious and unconscious levels. It took several weeks, but gradually he was able to connect with his genuine desire to help, and to offer counsel with more civility and compassion. Finally, all of the visitors had "moved on," even the hyper-conscientious Cantor Fitzgerald woman.

There is no clear evidence that Mike's dream of Connie's visitation and the freeing of his body from its suspension in a pre-pubescent state was directly linked to my attempt to adjust my conscious and unconscious observing lens in response to what was going on in the treatment. I believe, though, it is likely. As mentioned earlier, the nonlocal unconscious conveys its telepathic activity to our conscious mind in different dialects, some of which are more immediately understandable, while others require more effort to translate.

The telepathic events that are immediately recognizable, that satisfy our conscious minds' need for symmetry and clear data points, can be considered to be at one end of a continuum of telepathic communication, similar to the continuum ranging from transparency to opacity in dream symbolism. Others remain more elusive, more challenging to decipher, like a dream that leaves us with only partial pieces of a puzzle from which to draw a coherent, meaningful interpretation; yet it is no less a dream, and no less indicative of unconscious communication. There are several beautifully elaborated instances of what I call "first order" telepathic events elsewhere in this book, where two people can clearly connect the perceptions of one with very similar if not identical facts about the other. I will give just a brief example of one from my practice before describing another kind of telepathic communication from a different place on the continuum.

One of my patients, whom I'll call Gail, suffered from social anxiety and its resulting isolation. In our sessions, she had great difficulty even allowing thoughts and memories to come to mind. Often she declared that she had nothing to say because there were no thoughts in her head, and that I should tell her my thoughts. A few months into our sessions, Gail had a dream that she was in my kitchen and was surprised to see that there were bowls of apples all over the counter. In fact, I eat a lot of apples, and though I like other fruit as well, apples are my favorite, and for an odd sense of "security," I always make sure to have a couple bowls of apples, only apples, on my kitchen counter. When I told Gail of my apple "habit," I could tell that her "reaching" me in this way empowered her with a sense of agency, even pride, for which she had no model or encouragement from early childhood to adulthood.[2] Within a few weeks, she began to make connections between her social anxiety and the origins of the feelings of ostracism, inadequacy, and invisibility that had shaped her psyche.[3]

In the following case, I attempt to illustrate how the presence of telepathic communication may underlie many human interactions. Even if they are not identifiable by either party to the communication, they may have profound effects on each. To underscore this possibility, I return for a moment to the fact that what we can see, hear, touch, smell, and taste per second emerges from roughly 11 million bits of information per second that we receive and respond to, of which only a few enter our conscious awareness as something we see or hear or taste. If we accept the notion that our nonlocal unconscious consorts with far more information than is needed for our five senses, imagine how many millions of bits of unconsciously conveyed information our minds might be receiving per second, with only a tiny fraction reaching conscious awareness, and how varied the forms and symbols are in which this unconscious conveys the information it carries to our conscious mind.

Whose Garden Is It?

Bill came in for his initial session in a rage. He spent much of the time cursing and railing against the women in his life—his wife, coworkers, a neighbor. He told me that he had a hit list that consisted of several women, and then, looking at me with a sneer, wondered aloud if I might end up on that list. (He'd had great ambivalence about coming to see me and only did so because a much-admired male colleague had referred him.) As the session proceeded, and I listened to Bill's chronicling of how women had "done him wrong," a strange image flashed in my mind—an image of Bill, with a beatific smile on his face, digging in the soil of an elaborate, colorful flower garden. It seemed incongruous, to say the least, and I didn't pay much attention.

That evening, in thinking over Bill's session, I laughed to myself, assuming that my mind had produced the Bill-in-the-garden image as a comforting anchor for me to hold on to while listening to this rather scary man rant. Still, it seemed odd to me because gardening is not anything I've ever done, so it does not hold strong associations of comfort or security for me. In subsequent sessions, the weeks passed, the Bill-garden faded out of awareness; I believe that what had begun as a momentary surfacing of an image into conscious awareness became a subtle submerged detail that took residence in my psyche on an unconscious level.

I worked with Bill for over four years, during which time he developed trust in the analytic process and in me and made significant changes in some of his longstanding patterns, including those regarding his anger. And women. And then he moved upstate. About three years after I'd last seen him, I received a phone call from Bill. He was in Manhattan and wondered if I had a few minutes for him to stop by and say hello. I arranged the time, and Bill came to my office. After telling me about his new house, he took out his wallet, indicating that he had some pictures to show me. I assumed they might be of the house or of grandchildren. No—they were pictures of a large, strikingly beautiful flower garden. "This is my passion now," Bill said. "When I'm in my garden, I feel a kind of peace I never thought possible." And then he grinned, and said, "I bet this is the last thing you would ever have imagined me doing!"[4]

There are many ways of thinking about this uncanny unfolding of events. As we worked together, could the image of Bill in the garden, though residing mostly outside my conscious awareness, but definitely a part of my "observing instrument," have helped shape or awaken something in Bill's unconscious mind related to his own need for peace and beauty? Could a co-seeding of the garden have been initiated in our intersubjective field? Or, we could think of it within the framework of projective identification: As psychoanalyst Nathan Field (1991) suggested, "If we make the … assumption that we are not only separate but are also unconsciously connected, projective identification can be seen as the restoration of a vital, pre- existing condition" (p. 107). In Bill's case, because of a significant trauma he endured when he was nine, a trauma he had to navigate without support from his parents, he had developed a terse, tough, cynical style that lingered even after the tempering of his anger. It was clear to me that Bill had developed a disavowal and suppression of longings for anything resembling softness or gentleness, longings which could have been projected onto my receptive unconscious, conveyed to me in the form of the image of a sweetly smiling Bill in his garden. As psychoanalyst Nathan Field (1991) suggested: "If we make the … assumption that we are not only separate but are also unconsciously connected, projective identification can be seen as the restoration of a vital, preexisting condition" (p. 107). At very least, my unconscious holding of the peaceful garden image must have allowed me, without deliberate effort, to relate to Bill with more openness and affection than did many in his life, who were put off by his surface rage and bluster. The effect of this was most likely manifest in subtle facial expressions, tone of voice, and aspects of presence that may have been enough to awaken feelings in Bill that had been long buried. Of course, one could conclude that my image could have been a "simple" precognition of Bill in his future garden, or, as many might insist, it may have been mere coincidence. Either is possible, though neither of those ideas seem to hold the complexity, subtlety, and Moebius strip-like quality of mutual unconscious influencing that is the crucible of the healing alchemy of psychoanalysis. A question that arises for me when I think of this case: What if Bill had not come to visit me, had not shown me the garden photos? Would the flash image of Bill in the garden during that first session be considered a telepathic communication, even if the connecting "dots" were never revealed to either of us? In thinking about this, I am reminded of the well-known koan-like question: Does a tree falling in a forest make a sound if there is no one there to hear it? I think a crucial distinction between the seemingly unanswerable koan, and Bill's and my experience, may be that even an unrevealed telepathic (or precognitive telepathic) communication, one which never surfaces into conscious awareness of either of the two unwitting participants of the communication, may still initiate significant effects or changes in the psyches of both people at a fundamental level of an unmediated resonant space where there is no separation.[5]

Conclusion

It is becoming increasingly clear within a variety of academic fields that it is a fact of being human that we are simultaneously in relationship with both local, measurable and nonlocal, unbound dimensions of reality. The therapeutic encounter is representative of this characteristic of our nature: Just as there are no sharply delineated boundaries between patient and therapist in a co-created intersubjective field, there are no "fences" separating the space of the dyadic intersubjective field and the quantum-like field of infinite possibilities that surrounds and suffuses it (Rosenbaum, 2011, 2024).

Many contributors to this book have illuminated how telepathic incidents in psychodynamic therapy can enrich the relationship between therapist and patient and bring our attention to the "superordinate field" (Tennes, 2007, p. 510) that we participate in, often outside our conscious awareness. However, because these incidents occur infrequently in clinical practice, I think it is important to ask if and how acceptance of telepathy and its broader existential implications can inform clinical work outside of specific telepathic occurrences in treatment. I've suggested that a "telepathic principle" underlies and permeates our material existence, pointing to an unseen domain in which we are engaged in a shared space of communication whether or not such communication rises into conscious awareness. How might integrating this into our understanding of our own and our patients' lives and psyches change our perspectives and some of our theoretical assumptions? And, in turn, how might that change affect clinical work? At very least, we might listen with more discernment and curiosity when patients report certain experiences that may seem strange or even psychotic within a traditional framework.

The idea that "Freudian patients have Freudian dreams; Jungian patients have Jungian dreams, and so forth" (Hufford, 2003, p. 107) underscores the way in which our theoretical lenses impress their contours on a patient's unconscious. Consider, then, the potential effects of a theoretical lens that includes ongoing awareness on the nonlocal features of our experience, a lens that exists along with other theoretical perspectives, creating a kind of intrapsychic progressive lens. With subtle shifts of attention, this progressive lens can facilitate an ongoing awareness of both the data and interpretation-based analytic processes as well as the untrackable, unknowable dimension, the "O" of unexpected and unlimited possibilities that defy probabilistic projections regarding a patient's capacity for growth and change based on what is already known about them and their developmental history.

Seventy years ago, Balint (1955) wrote, referring to ESP in general: "Perhaps we analysts ought to accept the role of pioneers in this field," and he suggested that we relinquish "the professional hypocrisy … surrounding parapsychological phenomena" (p. 35).

Psychoanalytic work, with its immersion in unconscious processes, has always been a natural laboratory primed for the discovery of all sorts of derivatives of the nonlocal unconscious. If we can confront and overcome psychoanalysis's historically rooted fears (and our own individual fears) of being labeled irrational or indulging in "an infantile mode of thought" (Servadio, 1935, p. 210), and if we embrace telepathy and other forms of anomalous experience, we might recognize that we are uniquely well-positioned to contribute, with our abundance of "clinical facts" (Mayer, 1996), to a more nuanced understanding of the integration of the local (time-and-space-bound) and the nonlocal (unbound) aspects of our existence. As Balint's comment suggests, we should take our place on the front lines of exploring the complexity of our telepathic continuum and its far reaching implications alongside the physicists, neuroscientists, and philosophers who have ventured into this unfamiliar, paradigm-challenging territory.

Notes

1 It is important to note the distinctions between Jung's collective unconscious, Freud's timeless unconscious, and the nonlocal unconscious I present in this chapter. Though Jung's collective unconscious spans millions of years, back to our evolutionary beginnings, and universal archetypes resonate throughout time, they are, nevertheless, limited to the framework of human history. Regarding Freud's (1915) description of unconscious processes as timeless, and of the unconscious's permanent repository of memories bearing "no relation to time at all" (p. 135), these processes exist within an intrapsychic context and are bound by the history of the individual. In contrast, the nonlocal unconscious is more akin to a quantum-like field, and its domain extends beyond that of historical information or the accumulation of data points of past experience.

2 The need basis for psi was described by Ehrenwald (1978) who said that adults may retain telepathic capacity as a means of overcoming what he calls "communication gaps" (p. 22). Balint (1955), Schmeidler (1966) and others have noted that psi in analytic sessions may be prompted by a need on the part of the patient to break through the analyst's reserve, to cover the distance between them. As Balint described it: "Certain talented people solve this very strained situation by administering a therapeutic shock to their analyst by producing apparently parapsychological phenomena" (p. 33).

3 Self-disclosure is a much discussed topic in psychoanalysis—whether to, how much to and how to handle it in the treatment. With incidents of telepathy, there is a unique element added: The analyst has no choice in the material to be disclosed or not disclosed—the patient already "knows" and has unconsciously selected the details. The analysis of disclosure thus raises additional facets of countertransference, one example being how the analyst feels about being "found out." In this case, I'd been keenly aware of how unrecognized, invisible, and without recourse to be "seen" Gail felt in her childhood and in the present as well, and thought it appropriate to validate her capacity to initiate a connection and be responded to.

4 In this case, I did not disclose to Bill the image that had come to me in our first session, because I felt that would have been more about me, and that to do so would take away from his pride and ownership of the growth he'd achieved since we'd last met.
5 Portions of this section were previously published in Rosenbaum, R. (2011). Exploring the *other* dark continent: Parallels between psi phenomena and the psychotherapeutic process. *The Psychoanalytic Review, 98*(1), 57–90, DOI:10.1521/prev.2011.98.1.57.

References

Abbass, A. A., Hancock, J. T., Henderson, J., & Kisely, S. (2006). Short-term psychodynamic psychotherapies for common mental disorders. *The Cochrane Database of Systematic Reviews.* doi:10.1002/14651858.CD004687.pub3.

Atwood, G. E., & Stolorow, R. D. (1984). *Structures of subjectivity: Explorations in psychoanalytic phenomenology.* Atlantic Press.

Balint, M. (1955). Notes on parapsychology and parapsychological healing. *The International Journal of Psychoanalysis,* 36, 31–35.

Bion, W. (1995). *Attention and interpretation.* Jason Aronson.

Braud, W. G., & Schlitz, M. J. (1991). Consciousness interactions with remote biological systems: Anomalous intentionality effects. *Journal of Subtle Energies,* 2, 1–46.

Byrd, R. C. (1988). Positive therapeutic effects of intercessory prayer in a coronary care unit population. *Southern Medical Journal,* 81, 826–829.

de Beauregard, O. C. (1998). The paranormal is not excluded from physics. *Journal of Scientific Exploration,* 12, 315–320.

Driessen, E., Van, H. L., Don, F. J., Peen, J., Kool, S., Westra, D., Hendriksen, M., Schoevers, R. A., Cuijpers, P., Twisk, J. W., & Dekker, J. J. (2013). The efficacy of cognitive-behavioral therapy and psychodynamic therapy in the outpatient treatment of major depression: A randomized clinical trial. *The American Journal of Psychiatry,* 170, 1041–1050.

Ehrenwald, J.(1978). *The ESP Experience: A psychiatric validation.* Basic Books.

Ellis, G., & Silk, J. (2014). Scientific method: Defend the integrity of physics. *Nature,* 516, 321–323.

Field, N. (1991). Projective identification: Mechanism or mystery? *Journal of Analytical Psychology,* 36, 93–109.

Freud, S. (1920). *A general introduction to psychoanalysis.* Horace Liveright.

Freud, S. (1933/1953). Dreams and the occult. In G. Devereaux (Ed.), *Psychoanalysis and the occult* (pp. 87–90). International Universities Press.

Freud, S.(1963). The unconscious. In P.Reiff (Ed.), *General psychological theory: Papers on metapsychology*(pp. 116–150). Collier Books, Macmillan Publishing Company(original work published 1915).

Gallese, V. (2003). The manifold nature of interpersonal relations: The quest for a common mechanism. Philosophical transactions of the Royal Society of London. *Biological Sciences,* 358, 517–528.

Goldman, A. I., & Sripada, C. S. (2005). Simulationist models of face-based emotion recognition. *Cognition,* 94, 193–213.

Harris, W. S., Gowda, M., Kolb, J. W., Strychacz, C. P., Vacek, J. L., Jones, P. G., Forker, A., O'Keefe, J. H., & McCallister, B. D. (1999). A randomized, controlled trial of the effects of remote, intercessory prayer on outcomes in patients admitted to the coronary care unit. *Archives of Internal Medicine*, 159, 2273–2278.

Howard, D. (2009). Passion at a distance. In W. C. Myrvold & J. Christian (Eds.), *Quantum reality, relativistic causality, and closing the epistemic circle* (pp. 3–11). Springer.

Huber, D., Zimmermann, J., Henrich, G., & Klug, G. (2012). Comparison of cognitive-behaviour therapy with psychoanalytic and psychodynamic therapy for depressed patients: A three-year follow-up study. *Zeitschrift fur Psychosomatische Medizin und Psychotherapie*, 58, 299–316.

Hufford, D. J. (2003). Response. *Journal of Folklore Research*, 40, 99–109.

Jahn, R. G., & Dunne, B. J. (2007). A modular model of mind/matter manifestations (M5). *Explore*, 3, 311–345.

Jung, C. G. (1973). *Synchronicity: An acausal connecting principle* (R. F. C. Hull, Trans.). Princeton University Press (Original published 1952).

Lacan, J. (1991). *Freud's papers on technique, 1953–1954*. W. W. Norton.

Leichsenring, F., & Klein, S. (2014). Evidence for psychodynamic psychotherapy in specific mental disorders: A systematic review. *Psychoanalytic Psychotherapy*, 28, 4–32.

Leichsenring, F., Klein, S., & Salzer, S. (2014). The efficacy of psychodynamic psychotherapy in specific mental disorders: A 2013 update of empirical evidence. *Contemporary Psychoanalysis*, 50, 89–130.

LeShan, L. (1987). *The science of the paranormal: The last frontier*. The Aquarian Press.

Norretranders, T. (1998). *The user illusion: Cutting consciousness down to size*. Viking.

Rosenbaum, R. (2011). Exploring the other dark continent: Parallels between psi phenomena and psychotherapeutic process. *The Psychoanalytic Review*, 98(1), 57–90.

Rosenbaum, R.(2024). Psychoanalysis, psi phenomena, and spiritual space: Common ground. In L. J. Miller (Ed.), *The Oxford handbook of psychology and spirituality* (2nd ed., pp. 388–414). Oxford University Press. doi:10.1093/oxfordhb/9780190905538.013.17

Schmeidler, G.(1966). Two horns of a dilemma in relating ESP to personality. *Corrective Psychiatry and Social Therapy*, 12, 98–114.

Schmidt, S. (2012). Can we help just by good intentions? A meta-analysis of experiments on distant intention effects. *Journal of Alternative and Complementary Medicine*, 18, 529–533.

Servadio, E. (1935). Psychoanalysis and telepathy. In G. Deveraux (Ed.), *Psychoanalysis and the occult* (pp. 210–220). International Universities Press.

Shedler, J. (2010). The efficacy of psychodynamic psychotherapy. *The American Psychologist*, 65, 98–109.

Shedler, J. (2016). Where is the evidence for "evidence-based" therapy? *Journal of Psychological Therapies in Primary Care*, 4, 47–59.

Targ, R. (2019). What do we know about psi? The first decade of remote viewing research and operations at Stanford Research Institute. *Journal of Scientific Exploration*, 33(4). https://journalofscientificexploration.org/index.php/jse/article/view/1669

Tennes, M. (2007). Beyond intersubjectivity: The transpersonal dimension of the psychoanalytic encounter. *Contemporary Psychoanalysis*, 43, 505–525.

Turner, E. H., Matthews, A. M., Linardatos, E., Tell, R. A., & Rosenthal, R. (2008). Selective publication of antidepressant trials and its influence on apparent efficacy. *New England Journal of Medicine*, 358, 252–260.

Yakeley, J. (2014). Psychodynamic psychotherapy: Developing the evidence base. *Advances in Psychiatric Treatment*, 20, 269–279.

Chapter 9

When Our Hair Stands on End

Encounters with Non-Ordinary States

Karen Peoples

Karen Peoples, Ph.D., from the Psychoanalytic Institute of Northern California (PINC) in San Francisco believes that telepathic dreams between patient and analyst are "surprisingly common" and can occur so frequently for some individuals as to seem "quite ordinary." However, for Karen, the impact of shared similar dreams between her and her patient collided for her "with an electric shock," making her hair stand on end. She believes that telepathic occurrences often engender non-ordinary states of consciousness in the analyst, states that are markedly altered in contrast to ordinary ego awareness. Further she shows that these states exist across cultures and highlights the importance of expanding our clinical receptivity to and containment of pronounced state shifts in ourselves and in our patients. She proposes a psychoanalytic model of consciousness that places non-ordinary states on a normative spectrum from highly differentiated to highly undifferentiated, and identifies some of the neurological functions underlying psychic states along this spectrum.

* * * *

Psychoanalytic theory has evolved significantly from Freud's original one-person model, through a two-person intersubjective and relational model (Benjamin, 1988, 2013; Stolorow et al., 1994), and more recently to constructions about the analytic field itself as an intersubjective "third" influencing analyst and patient alike (Baranger & Baranger, 2008; Ogden, 2004; Stern, 2013a, 2013b). Going beyond this, Eshel (2006) writes of

> interconnectedness at a deep experiential-emotional level, which generates an emergent therapeutic entity that is fundamentally inseparable-into-its-two-participants. Hence, it is not a one- or two-person psychology, but a process whereby the two become an interconnected new entity or unit beyond their separate existences.
>
> (pp. 1604–1605)

Simultaneously, a crucial reconsideration in recent decades of actual external trauma as a significant pathogenic force has required a clinical reorientation

DOI: 10.4324/9781003611042-10

toward the effects, for example, of abusive family systems and the social surround on the developing mind of the child (Davies & Frawley, 1994; Herman, 1981, 1992). Infant research has likewise expanded psychoanalytic understanding of both healthy and disturbed interpersonal dynamics as they become internalized within the child's psyche and carried into adulthood (Stern, 1985; Beebe, 2018).

Recent theories of unconscious intergenerational transmission of trauma offer yet another angle on the importance of environmental factors in analytic practice (Auerhahn & Laub, 1984). The effects of social trauma from proximity to war, political upheaval, group dislocation, and ethnic or cultural discrimination have been linked to nonverbal and inchoate forms of mental disturbance, often triggering uncanny forms of unconscious communication (Davoine & Gaudilliere, 2004; Gurevitch, 2014). Reports of telepathic and other paranormal behavior indicate that they often co-occur with periods of increased social upheaval (Devereux, 1953). These expansions in analytic thinking evidence the permeability of the psyches of both patient and analyst and reflect the incorporation of the idea of a social unconscious into mainstream theory (Hopper, 2003). As a result, modifications in analytic technique have occurred: Namely, there is broad recognition by clinicians of the need to attend to unconscious derivatives from social and generational sources. Analyst Pichon-Rivière argued that "the individual and the group are illusions, derived from our mind's tendency to split and splinter complex wholes in order to be able to talk and think them through" (Tuber-Oaklander, 2011, p. 60).

Extending beyond the social unconscious, Bion (1970) contended that it is at-one-ment with the unconscious in its infinite, formless nature—what Bion called "O"—that enables the analyst to discover the emotional truth of the analytic moment. Grotstein (2000) notes that "O" "represents the ineffable, transcendental aspects of the mind, on one hand, and the raw proto-encounters or experiences that initially confront the mind, on the other" (p. xxxi). Following Bion, Eshel (2019a) presently argues for a "quantum psychoanalysis" that recognizes "a probabilistic, entangled realm of unity rather than division" (p. 267), necessitating the analyst's surrender to at-one-ment with "O" in order to reach the most inchoate forms of early patient trauma.

Despite all of these theoretical and clinical expansions, psychoanalytic thinking has yet to amend its core theories of psychic function to include uncanny forms of communication such as telepathy that challenge traditional conceptions of mind. Metapsychological models have yet to integrate the extensive body of clinical reports on telepathic communication that have been reported over the century (Evrard, 2024; Rabeyron, 2023; Rabeyron et al., 2021; Reichbart, 2024). Psychoanalyst Tennes (2022, 2024) has argued that a fear of the unknown, a fear of uncertainty, permeates the unconscious of the psychoanalytic endeavor itself, resulting in an over-reliance on rational interpretive modes and a theoretical devaluing of paranormal or non-ordinary states like telepathic dreams. Anxiety over the reputation of psychoanalysis led analysts like Ernest Jones (Eshel, 2006) and Ralph Greenson (Mayer, 2007) to caution against reporting telepathic incidents.

Telepathic Phenomena in Psychoanalysis

Rooted in Western, scientifically oriented culture, psychoanalysis has tended historically to privilege states of highly differentiated, symbolic cognition as a signature of psychic maturity. Telepathic communication strikes at the heart of this conception by erasing the separation and differentiation between minds, however briefly. Often occurring through dreams, telepathic phenomena can stimulate an altered state of consciousness in the perceiver, loosening the ego functions that normally operate to differentiate, categorize, and predict aspects of our environment, such as self-object awareness, judgment, and reality testing (Buchborn et al., 2023).

A number of analysts have observed how Freud (1921, 1922) was both fascinated by and conflicted about the paranormal phenomenon of telepathy throughout his life, frequently anxious that psychoanalysis would be tarnished by acknowledgement of it (Eshel, 2006; Mayer, 2007). He expressed disdain toward "occultists" who "will be ready to employ the methods of scientific enquiry only as a ladder to raise them over the head of science" (Freud, 1921, p. 180). Nonetheless, as psychoanalyst Reichbart (2019) states in his review of the history of telepathy in psychology and psychoanalysis:

> Freud did not consider telepathy unusual, rather he considered that it must be a common phenomenon. Too frequently, psychoanalysts who write in this area appear to have ignored this hypothesis by Freud. And all indications from the parapsychological field is that Freud was right.
> (p. 95)

Thus, the history of telepathic communication in psychoanalysis has been fraught (Cardeña, et. al, 2013; Evrard, 2024). Confusion—even alarm—about telepathy has likely contributed to its absence in analytic education and training. This volume is an effort to raise awareness of both the phenomenon and the controversy surrounding it, emerging from the 2024 IPTAR Conference, "A Century of Psychoanalytic Mystery: Telepathy in the Clinical Process." In this chapter, I discuss the way that the uncanniness of some telepathic experiences can give rise to what are called non-ordinary states of consciousness. I believe that the relationship between telepathy and non-ordinary states, which are often linked experientially, must be a part of this project. A comprehensive understanding of how these more extraordinary states of consciousness can arise within the normal spectrum of awareness is essential to prevent serious misunderstanding of patients. I argue that knowledge of non-ordinary states be integrated into our contemporary analytic models of the unconscious, and adjustments in technique occur for their fruitful containment within the transference/countertransference relationship.

First, I will highlight the way in which some telepathic experiences can generate a profound shift in the mental state of the perceiver—in this instance, the author—stimulating a non-ordinary state of consciousness (NOS's). Drawing from disciplines outside of psychoanalysis, I will then briefly illustrate how non-ordinary states of consciousness are widespread and highly valued across cultures and millennia of human history.

A Striking Clinical Encounter

Not all telepathic dreams evoke non-ordinary states. Some, however, are so striking that ordinary frames of reference as to who is the dreamer, and whose dream is being dreamt, can be upturned. When a telepathic dream triggers a non-ordinary state, as Tennes (2022) says, it is "like windows opening to a lived experience of self and other that, in its paradoxical, entangled fluidity … defies the fixity of our identifications in both time and space" (p. 15).

In my earlier life, I had experienced a number of uncanny and extraordinary states of consciousness through long-standing meditation and visualization practices. However, I was not prepared for the mind-altering state generated in me by the discovery of parallel dreams on the same night between myself and a patient. My early analytic training in child development had led to an internalization of the traditional analytic assumption that relatively undifferentiated states reflected a regression to early infant forms of consciousness. I held that belief until, some years ago, the following event occurred.

I was working with an emotionally constricted young physician in psychoanalytic psychotherapy. Although he had persisted in treatment doggedly for several years, I experienced him as quite passive and resistant. Progress seemed vexingly slow and frustrating. Interpretations of transference anxieties and of his underlying negativity in sessions were typically met with mild denials. The treatment only occasionally seemed to stir a ripple in his inner life, although he outwardly made gains in his career and resolved his schizoid tendencies sufficiently to marry.

During a familiar, rather lifeless period of the treatment, I dreamed one night that a rat was biting the connective tissue between my thumb and forefinger. I was in total darkness and the rat clung by its teeth to my hand, struggling. I felt a pang of fear anticipating an increasing sharpness to its bite, but I soon became aware that the rat was in a state of terror, writhing and flailing in panic. Realizing that the rat was clinging to my skin in fear for its life, I grew calmer. With my other hand I gently but securely took hold of its body and removed it, resolving my emotional tension, and the dream ended. The next morning the dream remained clearly in my mind. I reflected with curiosity on it, for the dream had touched me with a strange and tender feeling, but it disappeared from my mind as I went about my day.

In a session that afternoon with my reticent young physician, he told me a dream from the previous night: He was in total darkness and very frightened because a rat was biting the flesh between the thumb and forefinger of his hand. In escalating terror, he flung his hand wildly about, trying to dislodge the rat, to no avail. Suddenly, as he was being engulfed by panic, a hand came out of the darkness and removed the rat. Immensely relieved, my patient woke up.

As I listened to his tale, I could feel the hair standing up on my scalp and neck and could barely keep my jaw from dropping open. My skull felt too small for my mind. I was stunned not only by the fact that our dreams were nearly identical, but also and especially by the sudden, eerie feeling that we had been swept up by something much larger that commingled our psyches. Although very similar, our dreams held different intensities of affect and different forms of action. In my dream, I comprehended something of the rat's fear and helplessness, which enabled me to take action that restored safety for both myself and the frightened rat. For my patient, fear swept him into panic. It was as if his helpless desperation conjured help from "outside"—the hand reaching from the darkness to remove the rat. His dream, in its own right, was important but not exceptional. In parallel with my dream, it was startling and disorienting. Had his consciousness reached into my dreaming mind? Had mine reached into his? The feeling that we had interacted in each other's dreams and perhaps, thereby, altered their outcomes engendered an overwhelming experience of awe in me, awe that was not without a touch of terror.

Familiar interpretations occurred to me later about these dreams that seemed relevant and therapeutically useful. Most striking, however, was the dreams' uncanny doubling and intertwining on the same night. How are we to understand psychoanalytically the mechanism by which these kinds of unconscious transmission occur if we are implicitly bound to the preconception that consciousness resides within an individual mind? What do such occurrences intimate about the nature and function of consciousness as a whole? This startling experience suffused me with a quality of truth—a noetic experience—that I could not deny: namely, that the unconscious had a reach far more immense than the horizons I had glimpsed heretofore. It suddenly seemed to be a limitless presence much more encompassing, permeating, and awesome in its power than I had ever imagined. This uncanny encounter brought with it a realization that the unconscious dimension of the treatment constitutes a field in which proto-symbolic action and interaction are unfolding outside of the awareness of both patient and analyst. My limited, implicit preconception of the mind as a private, separate entity was irrevocably disrupted by this event.

Because of the overpowering nature of this experience that I struggled to contain in the session, something within left me feeling it was premature to share it with my patient, perhaps concerned that it might disassemble *him* as it threatened to do *me*. I regret to this day that I chose not to disclose it, because I think it could have provided powerful material for us to explore together. In particular, it would have enlightened us both as to how deeply connected we actually were.

Non-Ordinary States across Cultures

In response to our parallel dreams, I experienced what consciousness researchers call a non-ordinary state. Variously referred to as "anomalous," "paranormal," "altered," or "non-ordinary," they appear in the human record throughout the arc of history. Non-ordinary states are a markedly different state of consciousness from ordinary waking perception and brain function. They include shifts in the subjective sense of time, space, sense perception, physical boundaries, and—at times—a dissolution of the sense of a separate self. As noted consciousness researcher Charles Tart (1990) describes, these are not merely *quantitative* shifts in a single cognitive function such as arousal level, but rather "a qualitative alteration in the overall pattern of mental functioning such that the experiencer feels his consciousness is radically different from the 'normal' way it functions" (p. 13) (see also Cardeña et al., 2013; Cardeña et al., 2015).

I wish to distinguish telepathic communications per se from non-ordinary states. For some people, telepathic experiences are so frequent that they do not generate the significant state shift linked with NOS's. For example, psychoanalyst Janine de Peyer (2016) describes numerous unsettling instances of telepathic perception in a patient's dreams about her. Selectively disclosing the accuracy of some of her perceptions, de Peyer's patient remained quite unfazed. Her tendency to intuit very private information about her analyst that could not possibly be discerned otherwise was commonplace for the patient. The analyst, however, on at least one occasion of hearing what her patient knew about her private life, experienced an uncanny shift in which she "felt a strange loosening in my body, as if floating inside my skin" (p. 158). I consider this "floating" quality a state shift into non-ordinary consciousness.

Central characteristics of non-ordinary states were first described in Western psychology by William James (1982) and include: (1) ineffability; (2) noetic or revelatory truth quality; (3) transiency; and (4) passivity or surrender to the transformative power of the experience. NOS's appear in many forms, including hypnotic trance states, hallucinatory visions of both a personal and archetypal nature, significantly heightened or diminished sense perceptions, out-of-body experiences, synesthesia or the experience of one sense perception through another sense—such as smelling a color—paranormal experiences that strikingly alter consciousness, states of intense bliss, and significant changes in the sense of time and space in which consciousness seems to be "everywhere and nowhere" (Richards, 2016).

Non-ordinary states can be generated by sudden brain changes, as in the ecstatic insight that neuroanatomist Jill Taylor (2006) experienced in the midst of a massive stroke. They can also occur spontaneously through intense immersion in a work of art or a sudden uncanny moment of telepathic awareness. Commonly, NOS's are generated by extreme emotional or physical activation, through intensive meditation, through cultural rituals that induce a hypnotic-like trance such as praying, chanting, singing, or dancing, through the ingestion of psychedelic substances, through fasting, sleep- or sensory-deprivation, prolonged isolation, and so on. Neuroscientists suggest "[t]hese experiences presumably induce a state of relaxation that replaces fast brain activity in the front areas of the brain with slow wave activity representing more emotional information" (Winkelman, in Ember & Carolus, 2017).

Anthropological evidence for non-ordinary states exists in what are referred to as both spontaneous and "institutionalized" forms. Institutionalized forms refer to NOS's that are incorporated into cultural beliefs and practices. In one cross-cultural survey of 488 societies, 90% had some kind of cultural trance behavior or belief (Ember & Carolus, 2017). Below are a few examples of how ubiquitous these states are in humanity's collective history.

70,000–100,000 years ago at Blombos Cave in South Africa: Art motifs indicate the use of sensory deprivation and associated forms of visual hallucination.
1500 BCE to 1600 CE: Pre-Columbian Maya and Olmec peoples used hallucinogenic plants and toad venom to induce altered states.
4000–2000 BCE: Late Neolithic ceremonial complexes in Europe reveal art and artifacts thought to have been derived from hallucinatory imagery. Irish "passage tombs" are likely to have been designed as "multisensorial experiences" in which darkness and acoustic resonance could produce altered states of consciousness.
Prior to 1350 BCE: Pre-Incan sites in Bolivia and Peru show the use of mescaline in ceremonial circumstances.
1200 BCE–800 CE: Indo-European groups: Vessels were found that showed charred traces of cannabis sativa and sweet clover and were described by Greek historian Herodotus as part of a consciousness-altering repertoire for spiritual purification.

As cross-cultural researchers Ember and Carolus (2017) describe:

> These examples represent only a small fraction of the historical and archaeological evidence for institutionalized [non-ordinary states] …The ubiquity of these practices across time and space in human history suggests that [NOS's] play a fundamental role in the maintenance of human social fabric and human social–spiritual linkages.

In the West, non-ordinary states are under study in numerous research laboratories, in particular through the ways psychedelic agents stimulate neuronal activation in the brain similar to non-ordinary states triggered through other mediums, such as intensive meditation (Laukkonen & Slagter, 2021; Sacchet & Brewer, 2024). While NOS's are both markedly different from ordinary waking consciousness and do not occur in everyone, their ubiquity throughout history suggests that NOS's are both sought after and intrinsically interwoven within human culture.

Oceanic Experience in Psychoanalysis

In a non-ordinary state, normal ego functions temporarily "dissolve" or disappear into the background. On hearing my patient's dream so nearly identical to and seeming entwined in mine, I felt my consciousness expand and spread out in a remarkable, non-specific, but intensely charged way. When psychic boundaries and differentiating ego functions subside significantly beyond this, a sense of unity with the environment can occur. Such unitive states are fairly common in meditation and under the influence of psychedelics. In their written exchanges, Freud (1930) and Nobel laureate Romain Rolland described the subjective experience of such moments as "oceanic feeling … a feeling of an indissoluble bond, of being one with the external world as a whole" (p. 65). Although Freud was intrigued by such states, he admitted to having no experiences of oceanic feeling (Mayer, 2007). According to psychoanalyst Leavy (1995), studying the roots of unitive experience in the analytic literature, Freud refused to admit to the kind of "nonsensual, nonintellectual hold of reality" (p. 349) that oceanic states implied, asserting instead a genetic, developmental origin to them. In *Civilization and Its Discontents*, Freud (1930) commented:

> The idea of men's receiving an intimation of their connection with the world around them through an immediate feeling which is from the outset directed to that purpose sounds so strange and fits in so badly with the fabric of our psychology, that one is justified in attempting to discover a psychoanalytic—that is, genetic—explanation of such a feeling.
>
> (p. 65)

Following Freud, psychoanalytic thinkers have typically deemed this kind of undifferentiated state as reflecting psychotic, symbiotic, infantile, or otherwise "primitive" mental experience—that is, as either pathological or regressed (Fischman, 2019, 2023). This reductionistic tendency in analytic theory and practice fails to take into account non-pathological experiences that may reflect a transcending of ego-concerns and discovery of new, mature perspectives not heretofore glimpsed (Peoples, 2024; Peoples & Rundel, in press). Non-ordinary states of consciousness, which are typically marked by a high degree of undifferentiated mentation, have tended to remain unintegrated into the psychoanalytic canon. They remain largely unaddressed in mainstream analytic teaching, training, and supervision despite extensive curiosity about them. I suspect the majority of analytic training institutes continue to exclude attention to what psychoanalyst Elizabeth Lloyd Mayer (2007) called these forms of "extraordinary knowing."

When a telepathic communication triggers a non-ordinary state, it can generate a degree of astonishment that can both stun and flood one with awe, even terror. As Rilke (1978) perceptively commented: "Beauty is only the first touch of terror we can still bear, and it awes us so much because it so coolly disdains to destroy us" (p. 19). Non-ordinary states tend to threaten familiar dualistic perceptions of reality along with bedrock preconceptions of the separation between minds. They momentarily unravel our deeply rooted cognitive assumptions about a relatively linear developmental progression of increasing differentiation of self from object. Such unsettling experiences about ordinary reality can thus sorely undermine the sense of ego control by which we typically navigate an unpredictable world.

When psychoanalyst Mayer (2007) spoke to British analyst Adam Phillips about her strikingly uncanny experience in which a man with paranormal abilities precisely located the whereabouts of her daughter's beloved stolen harp, Phillips responded:

> Just consider it—the Oedipal taboo was nothing. Compared to the taboo invoked by *this quality of connectedness*—now *there's* a taboo! It suggests a capacity for connection that's far more fearful in implication than Oedipal love. It's far deeper, far more radical. Where are the boundaries? Where's Freud's concept of ego? It's overwhelming. Fascinating and full of promise but overwhelming.
>
> (p. 270, emphasis added)

The ambivalent interplay of fascination toward and fear of non-ordinary states continues in psychoanalysis, even though new windows on the subject have opened in recent years. French analytic researchers Evrard and Rabeyron (2012) documented over 100 analysts publishing on the topic of telepathy, starting with Freud. A handful of analysts, including Loewald (1972) and Milner (1952), have addressed the nature of unitive or timeless experiences (non-ordinary states), recognizing them as fundamental to the creative process. Loewald (1972) showed keen insight into the difference between a boundariless state of emptiness that engenders what he called "an experience of eternity" and a fragmented state of empty nothingness in which all sense of connection is lost—a state of unhealthy *de*differentiation. He noted:

> At one extreme is the experience of eternity where the flux of time is stayed or suspended ... where there is no division of past, present, and future, no remembering, no wish, no anticipation, *merely the complete absorption* in being ... All meaning is condensed in the undifferentiated, global unity of the abiding instant ... *and may flow out from there again to replenish the world of time with meaning*.
>
> (p. 405, emphasis added)

Loewald nodded to familiar analytic formulations of oneness states as a narcissistic defense, even as he attempted to preserve the experience as authentic. He concluded: "[Although] the experience of eternity may be best understood as a defense against anxiety, [that] does not invalidate it as a genuine *trans-temporal* state, a state that transcends time" (p. 405).

Marion Milner (1952), in describing the merging of the boundary in aesthetic experience, notes:

> the ability to tolerate a temporary loss of sense of self, a temporary giving up of the discriminating ego … perhaps requires a state of mind which has been described … as the aesthetic moment … In visual art the aesthetic moment is that fleeting instant, *so brief as to be almost timeless*, when the spectator is at one with the work of art he is looking at … He ceases to be his ordinary self, and the … aesthetic actuality is no longer outside himself. *The two become one entity; time and space are abolished* and the spectator is possessed by one awareness. When he recovers workaday consciousness it is as if he had been initiated into illuminating, formative mysteries.
>
> (p. 189, emphasis added)

I want to underscore how both Loewald and Milner recognized that these unitive states have transformative, generative qualities. Loewald saw them as "replenishing the world of time with meaning," and Milner saw experiences of oneness as "formative." In a chapter entitled "Why the Self Is, and Is Not, Empty" (Peoples, 2000), I likewise elaborated on this distinction between trans-temporal states of unitive awareness that *open out*, as it were, into oneness with "O" (Bion, 1970) from those states in which time is fragmented, leaving the dissociated psyche lost in the formless and catastrophic aloneness of the Real. Transcendent states of "emptiness" have a deeply restorative quality, releasing the individual from the preoccupations and obsessions of the ego.

Moments of oneness or unitive awareness entail a shift into a pronounced state of psychic *un*differentiation that is distinct from a dissociative or psychotic state of *de*differentiation. Consider an example of a unitive state in a patient with cancer who participated in a Johns Hopkins study on the effects of the psychedelic psilocybin:

> I had a sense of losing my observer. I no longer witnessed the images. I was becoming them … My body lit up, all parts in succession. It was the brightest thing I have ever seen. I glowed brilliantly from within … I felt I was being breathed or played like an instrument. Stunningly beautiful I got that every part of us is sacred. There is no speck of the cosmos which is apart from this breath.
>
> (Richards, 2016, p. 61)

This quality of profound connectedness, one that Adam Phillips exclaims is "far more fearful in implication than Oedipal love," speaks to both the fear of ego dissolution and the possibility of transcendent at-one-ment where love and faith intertwine in "O." Unitive experiences like the one above instill a *felt awareness* of profound interconnection, dissolving the layers of narcissism that cloud the mind and enshroud the heart (Peoples & Rundel, in press).

Contemporary neuroscience studies of non-ordinary states under psychedelics show changes in the Default Mode Network, an interconnected group of brain regions that are associated with introspective functions and internally directed thought, such as self-reflection and self-criticism. As individuals develop, pathways of neural activity in this and other brain regions are increasingly reinforced, and "quite literally come to constitute our 'default mode' of operating in the world, coloring the way we perceive reality" (Virdi, 2023). Psychiatrist Matthew Brown, a specialist in the treatment of OCD, likens overactivity in this brain network to experiences of "hypercriticality," "rigid thought patterns," and "automatic negative thought loops" about oneself (Virdi, 2023).

During the non-ordinary states of awareness stimulated by classic psychedelics like LSD, the Default Mode Network becomes relatively quiet (Swanson, 2018). Neuroscience researchers such as Robin Carhart-Harris (Kocarova et al., 2021) show that what transpires in such states is a "bottom-up" processing in the brain that loosens fixed narratives and patterns of thinking. This is akin, he says, to shaking the snow globe mentally (Pollan, 2018). Acute neuroplasticity in the brain occurs at these times, especially when supported therapeutically, leading to "an equanimous, open and psychologically flexible state of being which could be described as a recalibration of brain, mind and behavior, serving current and long-term psychological health" (Carhart-Harris et al., 2014). In psychoanalytic terms, non-ordinary states and the slower brain waves that typically accompany them tend to manifest in a fluid, liminal opportunity to transform these fixed patterns of conscious/unconscious action. This comports with one of the key aims of psychoanalysis, which is to facilitate the loosening of defenses that bind entrenched beliefs, allowing receptivity to new learning and thus new perspectives on self and life.

Summary

Psychoanalysis is rich with writings that chronicle patients' dreams and perceptions in which hair-raising details about the analyst appeared that the patient could not possibly have known, even in the age of Google. Attempting to make sense of her own striking experiences, Eshel (2006) drew on the Jungian conception of synchronicity as an "acausal connecting principle" in line with the idea of a "common subconscious" (pp. 1613–1614). This metapsychological speculation points to how our implicit concepts about the unconscious determine how we listen to—and hear—our patients. Is the unconscious of the patient a more-or-less boundaried sphere that interacts with the unconscious of the analyst only through phantasy projections and introjections? Is it a third subjectivity that is more than the separate unconscious minds of the dyad, as Ogden (2004) has written, or part of a dynamic field as Baranger and Baranger (2008) and Stern (2013a, 2013b) describe? Is it "beyond intersubjectivity," as Tennes (2007) suggests? Is it an infinite unconscious, as Bion asserted, in which our separate-seeming spheres of mind are perhaps but a protective illusion? Grotstein (2007) and Suchet (2016), in line with Bion, point to an ineffable and limitless unconscious that, in Suchet's terms, involves a "superconscious" that transcends the personal psyche in both its conscious and unconscious functions.

In a compelling 2021 article in *JAPA*, French psychoanalytic researchers Rabeyron, Evrard, and Massicotte attempt to integrate recent extensions in analytic theorizing that might account for telepathic transmissions between patient and analyst. Drawing on the work of Bion, Bolognini, Civitarese, and others, they suggest that "[t]hese theoretical contributions allow a greater understanding of transference at its most primary levels, that is, in a primary form of *fusion* in the *inter*psychic state" (p. 551, emphasis added). They add:

> The telepathic hypothesis leads us to question the most primary levels of symbolization and the profound nature of reality and suggest that certain interactions between analyst and analysand might transcend models of primary intersubjectivity, revealing something "beyond" intersubjectivity in the here and now.
>
> (p. 561)

The authors propose different levels in the stages of symbolization and conjecture that the most primary level—beyond and prior to symbolization—is where telepathic communication occurs. This "ontic" level would correspond to Bion's (1970) description of "O" and would be more primary than the mind's rudimentary formulation of pictograms, dreams, and verbal communication.

Valuable contributions such as these have been made toward a psychoanalytic metapsychology of telepathic communications and non-ordinary states. However, the use of words like "primary" tends to evoke very early developmental states in the analyst's mind. Going further in this direction, Rabeyron, Evrard, and Massicotte (2021) state that:

> [t]elepathy-like experiences would arise in this interpsychic state as a co-subjective relational mode giving rise to coalescence phenomena, the patient needing to *regress* to an undifferentiated and presubjective state in order to elaborate his or her experience.
>
> (p. 551, emphasis added)

Many cases of patient–analyst telepathic communication likely do arise from the patient's regression to primary, unrepresented experiences of infancy, generated by what analyst Eshel (2019a) describes as a "search engine" in the preverbal mind initiated by the uncontained effects of early trauma. However, the assumption of "regression to an undifferentiated and presubjective state" reasserts traditional analytic formulations that states of at-one-ment, union, or symbiosis are fundamentally infantile in nature. Eshel (2019b), whose cutting-edge work on telepathic communication I greatly admire, states "telepathic dreams impel us to go further, beyond projective identification, beyond intersubjectivity, into an enigmatic 'impossible' extreme of patient-analyst deep interconnectedness, at-one-ment, and unconscious communication in the analytic process" (p. 610). Yet, even as she argues for a "radical" psychoanalysis that embraces the idea of entangled psyches, Eshel consistently interprets her clinical accounts of telepathic experiences as stemming from infantile origins. The imposition of Freudian developmental concepts undermines and constrains her important metapsychological speculations. As I have hoped to underscore in this paper, the pull of Freudian notions of symbiosis and regression to infantile mental states as the primary explanation for telepathy doggedly persists within psychoanalysis.

I believe it is more accurate for psychoanalysis to incorporate a model of human consciousness that recognizes normal fluctuation, from infancy onward, between highly undifferentiated states to highly differentiated ones. This more accurately reflects what neuroscience is demonstrating about the brain and captures the richness and complexity of the human experience. Undifferentiated states likely predominate in early infancy, when the ego's nascent capacities for differentiation, categorization, and symbolization are gradually developing into higher order cognitive processes (Buchborn et al., 2023). For example, Winnicott (1965) highlighted the salutary effects of *un*integrated psychic states in the baby, distinguishing them from the disturbing experience of *dis*integration. He considered moments of unintegration as a nourishing experience, essential to the baby's "going on being."[1]

For the adult navigating a complex contemporary world, ordinary life typically requires that highly differentiated cognitive operations take precedence. However, as seen in the historical record and to the present day, cultures across the globe persistently engaged in activities that initiate highly undifferentiated states, including unitive or merger experiences. The desire to be transported by music, art, exhilarating activity, or, conversely, to quiet the activity of the ordinary mind through meditative practice is commonly sought in today's world.

Rethinking Analytic Models of Consciousness

The Freudian model of conscious, preconscious, and unconscious states has long dominated psychoanalytic theories of mind. The expansions noted at the beginning of this chapter that introduce a field theory of consciousness along with a social unconscious have gained widespread acknowledgment. Likewise, Bion's later work attesting to an infinite unrepressed dimension of the unconscious (distinct from the dimension in which psychic repression operates) has also been widely considered. In an effort to integrate Bion's work with the Freudian model, Belgian analyst Rudi Vermote (2021) distinguishes between the Freudian repressed unconscious, which he calls "psychic mind," and Bion's conception of the formless, "infinite," and unrepressed dimension of "O."

Vermote (2021) elaborates three modes of conscious/unconscious states that fluctuate on a continuum between finite and infinite, shifting back and forth from relative differentiation to relative undifferentiation. There are no clear boundaries between the three modes, but consciousness fluidly shifts between them. Each mode is characterized by different mental operations. Rational, discursive thought predominates in Mode One, shifting toward conscious/unconscious forms of knowing in Mode Two (Bion's "K," 1962), to at-one-ment with the formlessness and infinity of "O" in Mode Three. Vermote usefully identifies the technical approaches in clinical practice that correlate with and engage these three modes.

Like Milner and Loewald before him, Vermote (2021) speaks to the generative potential of at-one-ment with "O": "This infinite unrepresented and undifferentiated world, the largest part of the mind, is close to life. It is vitality!" (p. 4). Regrettably, like so many other analytic pioneers, Vermote labels this part of the human psyche "the infantile mind." While undifferentiation may be the ontological nature of mind in its origins in the newborn, I believe it is incorrect to consider this dimension only infantile in nature. Rather, following Grotstein (2000, 2007), I see the formless dimension of "O" as pre-existing and continuously present alongside psychic development.

Adult experiences of undifferentiation, such as the "aesthetic moment" Milner describes, entail a temporary but significant dissolution of ego boundaries. These can be formative in spurring psychic growth, but can also be transformative of deeply held beliefs. For the analyst to automatically conflate such experiences with infantile undifferentiated states risks collapsing reflection on the complex meanings that can occur for a patient. A patient can be left feeling profoundly misunderstood, the more transcendent aspects of their experience are foreclosed.

Despite his description of "O" as the infantile mind, Vermote's model is valuable because it elaborates states of consciousness that interact with, but are not reduced to, familiar analytic stages and phases of development (see Peoples & Rundel, 2025). Like Bion, Vermote (2021) sees this third mode holding "a deep healing potential and that we are only now beginning to see how this potential can be unleashed with our psychoanalytical device and technique" (p. 8). I strongly recommend that models of consciousness like Vermote's be incorporated in our analytic canon alongside our valuable understanding of psychic development.

Conclusion

The gaze in psychoanalysis ever-backward to earliest infancy exerts a powerful hold. It keeps us not merely *conceptually* bound, but it also keeps us *clinically* bound to potential misinterpretations of our patients' non-ordinary experiences, seeing them only as regressions rather than as potential expansions.[2] To ignore or reduce these experiences forecloses transformative possibilities for our patients. Investigating our implicit conceptual biases about these states and stepping, despite our fear, into the seemingly limitless mystery of the unconscious requires an expansion of our analytic receptivity in a way that may be unnerving, but which can only enhance our patients' ability to have faith in their own more formless states of being.

I believe our collective human ability to open to and tolerate porous, undifferentiated states of consciousness is as essential to strengthening psychic resilience, as is our capacity for rational thought. In psychoanalysis, the more we inform ourselves about—and allow ourselves access to—experiences like those that telepathic communication can stir, the more we can facilitate the psychic flexibility in ourselves and our patients that is indeed a hallmark of mental health.

For years, I vaguely imagined my unconscious as a semi-permeable sphere touching the edges of my patients' psychic spheres, sometimes interpenetrating in unsettling ways. But my patient's rat dream, arising on the same night "hand in hand," as it were, with my rat dream, palpably shook and rendered those imagined boundaries more permeable than I ever imagined. Telepathic communication, and the non-ordinary states they may stimulate, may indeed be evoked by unformulated infantile states of desperation, generating a psychic "search engine" that precipitates at-one-ment states between analyst and patient. I believe this was partially the case with my patient's rat dream, given his immense anxiety in the dream. However, telepathic communication may also represent a patient's expansion of consciousness brought on by a temporary, non-pathological dissolution of ego-identifications. Such transient dissolutions mark a signature non-ordinary state into undifferentiated fluidity within the unconscious that can open up crucial emotional truths and new perspectives for our patients on their inner and outer worlds.

In asking "Who is the dreamer, who dreams the dream?" James Grotstein (2000, 2007) directly addressed the ineffable reaches of consciousness, claiming: "Bion … launched a metapsychological revolution" in which he "perforated the flat world of Freud's and Klein's positivism … and introduced inner and outer cosmic uncertainty, infinity, relativism, and numinousness as its successor" (2007, p. 114). Grotstein (1998) spoke of an "ineffable Subject" within the individual in steady contact with this infinite field of consciousness. Similarly, in writing about the infinite nature of the unconscious, Brazilian analyst Leopold Nosek (2009) recognized how our concepts—our highly differentiated cognitive functions—"traumatize our objects." That is, they constrain our minds and thus our connection to the universe. Nosek, following the philosopher Levinas, urges analysts to welcome the unfamiliar terrain of the infinite *beyond* our concepts as we would a guest.

Extraordinary and yet so commonplace, non-ordinary states such as those initiated by telepathic communications appear to be intrinsically meaningful to and present in our human experience across cultures. They provide touchstones of deep interconnection that can carry the wounded heart and mind, through faith, back toward wholeness.

I can easily ascribe the dream of my rather stolid young physician to his unsymbolized, infantile dread as it provoked a desperate dream-cry for my containing alpha-function. As valid as this interpretation is, I feel it does not—and should not—preclude my simultaneous welcoming of the unconscious desire in both my patient and myself to be unleashed from our separate subjectivities into an uncanny communing, a dream-doubling in an uncanny—*unheimlich*—pocket of psychic time-and-space. Who is the dreamer who dreams the dream? Who, or what, is dreaming the dreamers?

Notes

1 Winnicott (1965) called it "unintegration," the infant's primary state of mind, and connected this with a state of "relaxation" in which the infant can take for granted the trustworthy holding of the mother such that no "need" to be integrated is experienced.

2 Infant researcher Daniel Stern (1985) strongly cautions clinicians not to conflate evidence from infant development with the psychological dynamics of adults.

References

Auerhahn, N. C., & Laub, D. (1984). Annihilation and restoration: Posttraumatic memory as pathway and obstacle to recovery. *International Review of Psychoanalysis*, 11, 327–344.

Baranger, M., & Baranger, W. (2008). The analytic situation as a dynamic field. *International Journal of Psychoanalysis*, 89, 795–826.

Beebe, B. (2018). My journey in infant research and psychoanalysis: Microanalysis, a social microscope. In S. Lord (Ed.), *Moments of meeting in psychoanalysis: Interaction and change in the therapeutic encounter* (pp. 13–44). Routledge. doi:10.4324/9781315389967-2.

Benjamin, J. (1988). *The bonds of love: Psychoanalysis, feminism, and the problem of domination*. Pantheon.

Benjamin, J. (2013). The bonds of love: Looking backward. *Studies in Gender and Sexuality*, 14, 1–15.

Bion, W. R. (1962). *Learning from experience*. Karnac.

Bion, W. R. (1970). *Attention and interpretation*. Karnac.

Buchborn, T., Kettner, H. S., Kärtner, L., & Meinhardt, M. W. (2023). The ego in psychedelic drug action: Ego defenses, ego boundaries, and the therapeutic role of regression. *Frontiers in Neuroscience*. Retrieved from www.frontiersin.org/journals/neuroscience/articles/10.3389/fnins.2023.1232459/full.

Cardeña, E., Lynn, S. J., & Krippner, S. (Eds.) (2013). *Varieties of anomalous experience: Examining the scientific evidence, second edition*. American Psychological Association.

Cardeña, E., Palmer, J., & Marcusson-Clavertz, D. (Eds.) (2015). *Parapsychology: A handbook for the 21st century*. McFarland.

Carhart-Harris, R. L., Leech, R., Hellyer, P. J., Shanahan, M., Feilding, A., Tagliazucchi, E., Chialvo, D. R., & Nutt, D. (2014). The entropic brain: A theory of conscious states informed by neuroimaging research with psychedelic drugs. *Frontiers of Human Neuroscience*. Retrieved from www.frontiersin.org/journals/human-neuroscience/articles/10.3389/fnhum.2014.00020/full.

Davies, J. M., & Frawley, M. G. (1994). *Treating the adult survivor of childhood sexual abuse: A psychoanalytic perspective*. Basic Books.

Davoine, F., & Gaudilliere, J-M. (2004). *History beyond trauma: Whereof one cannot speak, thereof one cannot stay silent*. Other Press.

Devereux, G. (Ed.). (1953). *Psychoanalysis and the occult*. International Universities Press.

de Peyer, J. (2016). Uncanny communication and the porous mind. *Psychoanalytic Dialogues*, 26, 156–174.

Ember, C. R., & Carolus, C. (2017). Altered states of consciousness. Retrieved from https://hraf.yale.edu/ehc/summaries/altered-states-of-consciousness.

Eshel, O. (2006). Where are you, my beloved: On absence, loss, and the enigma of telepathic dreams. *International Journal of Psychoanalysis*, 87, 1603–1627.

Eshel, O. (2019a). *The emergence of analytic oneness: Into the heart of psychoanalysis*. Routledge.

Eshel, O. (2019b). Would clinical psychoanalysis shy away from delving further into the unknown? On the mystery of telepathic dreams. *International Journal of Psychoanalysis*, 100, 608–610.

Evrard, R. (2024). Parapsychology explained to psychoanalysts: A guide for my misinformed colleagues. Paper presented at the IPTAR Conference,A Century of Psychoanalytic Mystery: Telepathy in the Clinical Process, New York.

Evrard, R., & Rabeyron, T. (2012). Les psychanalystes et le transfert de pensée: Enjeux historiques et actuels. *L'Evolution Psychiatrique*, 77, 589–598.

Fischman, L. (2019). Seeing without self: Discovering new meaning with psychedelic-assisted psychotherapy. *Neuropsychoanalysis*, 21, 53–78.

Fischman, L. (2023). Psychedelic-assisted psychotherapy in 3-D: Acceptance, connectedness, and defensiveness. *Neuropsychoanalysis*, 25, 217–236.

Freud, S. (1921). Psychoanalysis and telepathy. In J. Strachey (Ed. & Trans.), *The standard edition of the complete psychological works of Sigmund Freud* (Vol. 18, pp. 173–194). Hogarth Press.

Freud, S. (1922). Dreams and telepathy. In J. Strachey (Ed. & Trans.), *The standard edition of the complete psychological works of Sigmund Freud* (Vol. 18, pp. 197–220). Hogarth Press.

Freud, S. (1930). Civilization and its discontents. In J. Strachey (Ed. & Trans.), *The standard edition of the complete psychological works of Sigmund Freud* (Vol. 21, pp. 57–146). Hogarth Press.

Grotstein, J. (1998). The numinous and immanent nature of the psychoanalytic Subject. *Journal of Analytical Psychology*, 43, 41–68.
Grotstein, J. (2000). *Who is the dreamer, who dreams the dream?*The Analytic Press.
Grotstein, J. (2007). *A beam of intense darkness.* Karnac.
Gurevich, H. (2014). *The language of absence and the language of tenderness: Therapeutic transformation of early psychic trauma and dissociation as resolution of the "Identification with the aggressor"*. Paper presented to the San Francisco Center for Psychoanalysis.
Herman, J. (1981). *Father–daughter incest*. Harvard College.
Herman, J. (1992). *Trauma and recovery: The aftermath of violence—from domestic abuse to political terror.* Basic Books.
Hopper, E. (2003). *The social unconscious: Selected papers.* Jessica Kingsley Publishers.
James, W. (1982). *The varieties of religious experience: A study in human nature.* Penguin.
Kocarova, R., Horacek, J., & Carhart-Harris, R. (2021). Does psychedelic therapy have a transdiagnostic action and prophylactic potential? *Frontiers in Psychiatry.* Retrieved from www.frontiersin.org/journals/psychiatry/articles/10.3389/fpsyt.2021.661233/full.
Laukkonen, R., & Slagter, H. (2021). From many to (n)one: Meditation and the plasticity of the predictive mind. *Neuroscience & Biobehavioral Reviews*, 28, 199–217.
Leavy, S. A. (1995). Roots of unitive experience. *Psychoanalytic Review*, 82, 349–370.
Loewald, H. (1972). The experience of time. *Psychoanalytic Study of the Child*, 27, 401–410.
Mayer, E. L. (2007). *Extraordinary knowing*. Bantam.
Milner, M. (1952). Aspects of symbolism in comprehension of the not-self. *International Journal of Psychoanalysis*, 33, 181–194.
Nosek, L. (2009). Body and infinite: Notes for a theory of genitality. Paper presented at the 46th IPA Congress, Psychoanalytic Practice: Convergences and Divergences, Chicago.
Ogden, T. H. (2004). The analytic third: Implications for psychoanalytic theory and technique. *Psychoanalytic Quarterly*, 73, 167–195.
Peoples, K. (2000). Why the self is, and is not, empty: Traumatic and transcendent forms of emptiness. In A. Elliott & C. Spezzano (Eds.), *Psychoanalysis at its limits: Navigating the postmodern turn* (pp. 239–269). Free Association Books.
Peoples, K. (2024). The mystery of the unconscious: Non-ordinary states in psychedelic-assisted therapy. In J. A. Butler, G. Herzberg & R. L. Miller (Eds.), *Integral psychedelic therapy: The non-ordinary art of psychospiritual healing* (pp. 174–202). Routledge.
Peoples, K. & Rundel, M. (2025). Expansion and regression in oceanic experience: A model of psychedelic consciousness for psychoanalysis. *Psychoanalytic Dialogues*, 35(6), 808–830.
Pollan, M. (2018). *How to change your mind.* Penguin Press.
Rabeyron, T. (2023). *Codex anomalia: De l'énigme du psi à la relation psyché-matière.* InterEditions.
Rabeyron, T., Evrard, R., & Massicotte, C. (2021). Psychoanalysis and telepathic processes. *Journal of the American Psychoanalytic Association*, 69, 535–571.
Reichbart, R. (2019). *The paranormal surrounds us: Psychic phenomena in literature, culture and psychoanalysis.* McFarland.

Reichbart, R. (2024). Discussion of Janine de Peyer's "Piercing the veil: From intiuition to telepathic receptivity. Paper presented at the IPTAR ConferenceA Century of Psychoanalytic Mystery: Telepathy in the Clinical Process, New York.

Richards, W. (2016). *Sacred knowledge: Psychedelics and religious experiences.* Columbia University Press.

Rilke, R. M. (1978). *The Duino elegies.* Norton & Co.

Sacchet, M. D., & Brewer, J. A. (2024). Advanced meditation alters consciousness and our basic sense of self. *Scientific American.* Retrieved from www.scientificamerican.com/article/advanced-meditation-alters-consciousness-and-our-basic-sense-of-self/.

Stern, D. B. (2013a). Field theory in psychoanalysis, part 1: Harry Stack Sullivan and Madeleine and Willy Baranger. *Psychoanalytic Dialogues*, 23, 487–501.

Stern, D. B. (2013b). Field theory in psychoanalysis, part 2: Bionian field theory and contemporary interpersonal/relational psychoanalysis. *Psychoanalytic Dialogues*, 23, 630–645.

Stern, D. N. (1985). *The interpersonal world of the infant: A view from psychoanalysis and developmental psychology.* Basic Books.

Stolorow, R., Atwood, G., & Brandchaft, B. (Eds.). (1994). *The intersubjective perspective.* Jason Aronson.

Suchet, M. (2016). Surrender, transformation, and transcendence. *Psychoanalytic Dialogues*, 26, 747–760.

Swanson, L. R. (2018). Unifying theories of psychedelic drug effects. *Frontiers in Pharmacology.* Retrieved from www.frontiersin.org/journals/pharmacology/articles/10.3389/fphar.2018.00172/full.

Tart, C. T. (1990). *Altered states of consciousness.* Dutton.

Taylor, J. B. (2006). *My stroke of insight: A brain scientist's personal journey.* Plume.

Tennes, M. (2007). Beyond intersubjectivity: The transpersonal dimension of the psychoanalytic encounter. *Contemporary Psychoanalysis*, 43, 505–525.

Tennes, M. (2022). On revisiting Stoller's telepathic dreams. Paper presented at the Annual Stoller Lecture, New Center for Psychoanalysis, Los Angeles.

Tennes, M. (2024). *Discussion of Ofra Eshel's "Where are you, my beloved?"* Paper presented at the IPTAR ConferenceA Century of Psychoanalytic Mystery: Telepathy in the Clinical Process, New York.

Tuber-Oaklander, J. (2011). Enrique Pinchon-Rivière: The social unconscious in the Latin American tradition of group analysis. In E. Hopper & H. Weinberg (Eds.), *The social unconscious in persons, groups and societies: Mainly theory* (pp. 45–68). Routledge.

Vermote, R. (2021). The infantile mind. Paper presented at the Biannual Congress of the International Psychoanalytic Association.

Virdi, J. (2023). Psychedelics and the default mode network. *Psychedelics Today.* Retrieved from https://psychedelicstoday.com/2020/02/04/psychedelics-and-the-default-mode-network/.

Winnicott, D. W. (1965). Ego integration in child development. In *The maturational processes and the facilitating environment: Studies in the theory of emotional development* (pp. 56–63). International Universities Press.

Chapter 10

Telepathic Communications in Dreams and in the Psychoanalytic Process

Who Creates Them, and How Do They Happen?

Fonya Helm

Fonya Helm, Ph.D., is from the Contemporary Freudian Society (CFS) and practices in Virginia Beach, Virginia. She recounts here the intimate working through of her relationship to a female patient in which telepathy became a mutual part of their interaction and its existence served to draw them closer together. It began when the patient telepathically picked up on details of Fonya's a new house which included the new consulting room to which Fonya was to move. In a dream, the patient picked up on the appearance of the new house and the grounds, and also on a difficulty that Fonya and her husband were having with the contractor. Later, a second telepathic non-dreaming event took place with the patient concerning Fonya's health. This patient's early developmental history, as with Ofra's patients, involved maternal absence and Fonya explores the extent to which this desire helped to construct aspects of the dream. To a greater extent than in some other accounts, Fonya brought into the open the patient's tendency toward telepathy and during the treatment, they spoke about it with each other. In addition, Fonya explores the telepathic studies and thoughts of a variety of other psychologists and psychoanalysts including Montague Ullman and Stanley Krippner, Richard Reichbart, Elizabeth Lloyd Mayer, and Rupert Sheldrake.

* * * *

The Telepathic Dream

My patient and I decided to present the dream as she remembered it, then discuss how our perception and knowledge of the dream changed as time went by, as part of the psychoanalytic process of our work together. The treatment has been lengthy and is ongoing.

Her dream took place many years ago when I was planning to move to Virginia, hours away by car from where I had been living and working. My plan was to continue my work via Skype and phone, and I told her

DOI: 10.4324/9781003611042-11

approximately two years ahead, so we both would have plenty of time to assimilate this challenging change. During the first year before we moved, my husband and I had purchased our new home with an office and were building a large porch along the back of the house.

Her first report of the dream took place during this period in my home office, which was in a stone Tudor house that had a *large screened porch* on the second floor. She could see this porch by looking up as she walked down the stairs onto the patio in the back of the house to get to the waiting room. At the back of the house, there also was a steep slope with tall leafy trees in the summer, but bare in the winter, making a large body of water very visible.

This dream occurred during a session several months after I had told her I was planning to move. Here is the dream, reported in her words, as best as she and I can remember:

> I was at your new house and the backyard of the house was kind of like it is here and it sloped down toward water. But this slope was gentle and there were hardly any trees. I was in the backyard lying down in the grass near a small lake. I didn't want you to see me. I was looking up at the porch, hiding and feeling embarrassed about being intrusive. I was trying to get to the other side of the yard, before you saw me.

Surprised and startled, I told her how interested I was in the accuracy of her description of the land at the new house with its gentle slope, mostly grass and only a few trees. I felt pleased, and I told her what she said was accurate in her description of the land and the water. I also said she would be able to see for herself when she was able to visit the new office that also would be in my home. I felt somewhat apprehensive and not entirely comfortable as I was telling her about the new place, since self-disclosure of any information by the psychoanalyst was considered a boundary crossing, if not a boundary violation, by many other practitioners at that time. I listened very carefully for her response and was relieved that she received the information very well, although she said she felt somewhat uncomfortable about knowing the information and she did not want anyone to think she had "special powers." She did not elaborate, and I did not address the issue of the "special powers," feeling unsure about how to approach it.

I also did not tell her that my husband and I were having a second-floor porch built, another *large screened porch* about the same size as the one in the house where she was already was coming for her treatment.

From time to time in our work, we talked about the dream, and she would describe it in more detail. This dream was different from her usual dreams in that the grass was greener—very green—and it all seemed very real. She thought she had been telepathic and still felt somewhat embarrassed.

When she finally came to my office in the new home more than a year later, she initially was disappointed because nothing in the front of the house or near the side entrance of the waiting room looked anything like what she had seen in her dream. But when I took her around to the back of the house, she was excited about her accuracy of the details of the water, trees, and slope of the land. She said the land sloped down to the water at just the right angle, and the trees looked just the way they did in her dream. *The porch, however, did not*. The porch was a different color, and she could see it had screens. In her dream, there were no screens. The posts that held up the roof also looked different; they had different-sized spaces between them.

I was especially interested in these errors about the way the porch looked and wondered what could have caused the difference between her very accurate picture of the land, the water, and the number of trees, and her inaccurate perception of the porch. After all, she had created the dream, drawing on something in my mind, I thought. That would be the knowledge that I had about the building of the porch and what the backyard looked like—knowledge that I had not shared with her. I knew also that the dream had to be related to the enormous change in our work to Skype and phone that was ahead of us. The dream was about us, our relationship, and the upcoming loss of our physical workspace and the view she saw every day.

I also knew that she had learned that I had a husband, and I began to think more about that. Initially, I had the intuition that her hiding in the grass, feeling embarrassed about not wanting to be seen, might have had something to do with him. Over the years between the dream and now, we had talked often about the dream, and I began to notice that often we both "forgot" that part of the dream. We had been focused on her dream's accurate depiction of the land, trees, water—the natural world—and the distortions in how the completed porch actually looked when she eventually came to my new office.

I realized my husband also could have been part of the "surround" that created the information, the surround that Richard Reichbart (2019) discussed in his book *The Paranormal Surrounds Us*. Reichbart notes that when

> things telepathic occur in the clinical setting, it often is not just as a one-way or even as a two-way street between patient and analyst or between two patients but it [is] as if a "telepathic surround" has been established, which can draw in a number of people … It is almost as if [there is] a search engine that focuses on an issue or an anxiety, an event or a symbol, and then taps people associated unconsciously with each other. (pp. 111–112)

I then began to think about how many people might have been involved in a "surround" of anxiety and strong feelings about the porch, similar strong feelings that could somehow transmit the different images each had of how the porch was going to look when it was completely finished. In Reichbart's description of a "surround" created by different patients with different ideas, but similar strong feelings about wanting to be included, he adds,

> [T]he psychoanalyst's anxiety experiences may be brought parapsychologically to a patient's dream, or to a patient's associations, or even to another patient's similar experiences, and then a third or fourth patient may also in effect unconsciously participate, as if those patients too unconsciously desire attention from the analyst and want to be included. (p. 112)

Many People Could Have Contributed to the Formation of the Dream

When my patient had the dream—more than a year before the move—the porch was still being built, so it was not held in mind by anyone in a fully complete way. The contractor was a nephew of one of our new neighbors, who had highly recommended him. The contractor and my husband shook hands and agreed on a plan to build the porch. About five men who were going to help build the porch were also present and, in retrospect, I remember feeling uneasy and disliking them for what seemed like a peculiar contemptuous attitude. The contractor himself seemed friendly.

We expected the contractor to mail us a contract, but he did not do so, and he kept making excuses when we inquired about it. He began building the porch without a contract, and he sent bills without any details about what he was doing. We then discovered he had lied and was grossly overcharging us. I stopped paying his bills, and he sued us. His workers stopped working before completely finishing the porch, without cleaning everything up completely, but it was structurally completed and painted.

During this time, in the middle of this swirl of upset, anger and disappointment felt by so many in the "surround" of the analytic work my patient and I were doing together, my patient had the dream. Perhaps so many conflicting emotions and images about how the porch looked could have made it harder for her to get accurate information about the porch. The land and the water were not being constructed or landscaped, and they had not changed, so it might have been easier to gain information about them, since they were being held in mind peacefully in comparison to the upset about what was going on with the porch. Fast forward to the end of the story: My husband found a very kind mediator and former builder who was very helpful and testified for us; we basically won the mediation, but the contractor was allowed to overcharge somewhat, so relative peace was restored.

I strongly felt my relationship with the patient deepened when I showed her the backyard with mostly green grass and only a few trees sloping down to the water. My patient shares my feeling that our relationship deepened at that time, when she could walk around freely, then turn around to look up at the porch, and discuss it with me. Our discussions had always seemed to deepen our connection and had a calming effect on us both, but now I noticed how much easier it had become for her to trust me, feel more included and less worried about being abandoned, a major issue since the beginning of our work.

I knew from the beginning of our work that her fear of abandonment had begun early in her life, because of something she said to me during our first few sessions. She said, "Nothing happened to me before the age of five," and I knew that plenty had happened.

For years, though, I didn't hear about anything, as she was telling me about many later experiences and feelings that were extremely important, so the work we did on the earlier experiences took place only through the unconscious connections with the later experiences we actually talked about. No words were available yet.

Gradually, I found out more information about her early life, but it was only years later when I was astounded by Ofra Eshel's work and what she had discovered about her patients that I realized how important some of the information was. I learned that Eshel had five patients who had telepathic ability, and all of their mothers except one had partners who were away from the mother and the baby for long stretches of time during the patient's infancy.

These are the "mothers who were absent within absence." These mothers were physically present but emotionally absent and disconnected, due to the absence of the husband/father. My patient's mother was without her husband for the first six months of my patient's life.

I had already seen a picture of my patient when she was a baby six months old sitting on her mother's lap. Her mother was holding her, and they both were facing the camera. She was a beautiful baby and looked alert, observant, and fully present. Her mother, though, had a vacant look, as if she were detached and a part of her had gone somewhere else. I was concerned about the vacant look, and I had a strong feeling that something might be seriously wrong with the mother's ability to connect and be fully present with her baby.

Years later, I realized that this situation might have something to do with my patient's ability to develop her telepathic ability. My patient was very sensitive to extremely slight sounds—unusually so. I have wondered if she began listening for very slight sounds when she had to wait in her crib for her mother, who now had three young children and no one else to help. It would make sense if her mother had to be busy taking care of three children, including two active boys. Listening to her older brothers playing together and other family activities, while she waited for her turn for her mother's attention in her crib, could have helped to begin sharpening her listening skills. By the time she was an adolescent, she had had other opportunities to develop the outstanding listening skills she now has as an adult.

As an older child, my patient remembered rubbing her sheet before she went to sleep and, from time to time, some years after she had seen the porch, I heard her rubbing a sheet when we had a phone session. It comforted her and soothed her, but I always felt slightly perturbed, on the alert, as if she might be angry and frustrated, since she wanted something that wasn't available to her.

Perhaps her rubbing a sheet and my idea of a bed might relate to the part of the dream that she and I often "forgot" to include when we talked about the dream: "I was in the backyard lying down in the grass near a small lake. I didn't want you to see me and I was trying to get to the other side of the yard while staying low to the ground." In the dream, she was feeling embarrassed and wanting to hide. When we eventually talked in some detail about her embarrassment, I became more aware of her curiosity and assertiveness, and I felt somewhat uncomfortable and intruded on. I thought she must have been curious about my husband and me. She had grown up in a part of the country where second floor porches often were used as sleeping porches, and I wondered if she imagined my husband and I slept on the porch. It was a big porch, definitely big enough for a bed and other furniture. I felt while she wanted very much to be included, she also felt guilty and embarrassed about intruding into our personal space and perhaps struggled with excitement about loving and sexual feelings she did not discuss. Nonetheless, she was assertive and curious, supporting Janine de Peyer's finding of the analysand's curiosity about the analyst's personal life: Intrusiveness and aggression can be part of telepathic communication.

As we think about the dream and both the accurate and inaccurate parts of the telepathic communication, we can see the influence not only of the patient and the analyst, but also the influence of the other people who were connected to the analyst and had a strong emotional involvement. We also see the influence of both loving and assertive feelings as part of this emotional involvement.

Each time my patient and I have talked about her telepathic dream experiences, our relationship deepened, making her feel more comfortable and safer with me and making it possible for me to learn more, something I like very much. Most important for her feeling of safety and acceptance was the time she came to my new home office, and I showed her around, so she could see for herself the slope of the land, the trees, and the porch. This experience was especially meaningful for both of us. Showing her around was definitely an unusual way for a psychoanalyst to behave, but the overall effect was very good.

The Largest, Most Successful Study of Telepathic Dreaming

This study was done by Montague Ullman, M.D. and Stanley Krippner, Ph.D. in the 1960s at Maimonides Medical Center at City College of New York, and it took place over a period of ten years. My description also will introduce a researcher whose work I want to mention as a way to begin to think about what might be involved in telepathic transmission of unexpected knowledge.

Strong emotion is present in most reports of telepathic dreams, and it was found regularly in this study. Ullman and Krippner used a new indicator of dreaming that had been discovered ten years earlier in 1953 called Rapid Eye Movement (REM) sleep. They monitored the dreamers to discover when their eyes were moving under their closed eyelids and when they were beginning a dream.

In the meantime, a student in another room, who knew nothing about the purpose of the study, was alerted by a buzzer when the dreamer went into REM sleep. At that time, the student tried to send a visual image of a picture that was in a sealed envelope. The picture had been randomly selected before from a group of 25 pictures. After the dream was over, the researchers woke up the dreamer to ask questions about the dream. They woke the dreamers up three or four times a night, each time REM sleep ended, and made transcripts of each dream. Three independent judges read the transcripts and matched the visual images in the dream to the pictures from the large group that fit best with the dreams. Over 450 trials, during six years, the judges chose the correct targets enough times so the odds of choosing them by chance were 1 in 75,000,000 (Mayer, 2007). One of the findings was that strong emotion was present during telepathic dreaming. Another finding was that telepathic dreams had errors in them, just like my patient's dream did. It was not always easy to match them with the pictures.

Telepathic Dreams Follow Rules of Dream Construction

Sixty years earlier, Freud had already begun to discover both the presence of strong emotion and the errors that would be expected to occur in telepathic dreams, since they turned out to follow the rules of dream construction described in *The Interpretation of Dreams* (1953, original work published in 1899) and in the papers that he wrote in the 1920s about telepathy but never published in his lifetime. Reichbart (this volume) discusses Freud's examples of how telepathic dreams follow what Freud discovered about these rules. Very early in his work, Freud had discovered condensation, displacement, and other means of representation, constructed during the day and used for dreaming.

Freud considered *The Interpretation of Dreams* his best work. He emphasized strong emotion is one of the most important features of dreams, and later stated strong emotion is also there in telepathic dreams. He did his own studies of telepathic dreaming with Ferenczi, Jung, and sometimes his daughter, Anna, but did not publish them.

How Might Strong Emotion Facilitate Telepathic Transfer of Information?

Back to the 1960s telepathic dream study. Krippner noted that strong emotion was often present, and he also thought something else was going on to help facilitate the telepathic transfer of emotion connected with important information. He was interested in finding out if sunspots or phases of the moon were important. He asked Michael Persinger, a young psychologist, to correlate the data of telepathic successes with known sunspots and other activity of the global electromagnetic field. Persinger found greater telepathic success on the calmer nights, the nights with less activity. Those nights had fewer electrical storms and fewer sunspots.

Persinger went on to become a professor at Laurentian University in Sudbury, Ontario in Canada, where he spent his whole career studying low level electromagnetic fields in plants, fish, and mammals, including people. By the time he passed away in 2018, he had published more than 500 papers in peer-reviewed journals. In the studies with people, he and his colleagues embedded low-level local electromagnetic fields with signals like those emitted by our amygdala and hippocampus, two structures in our limbic system, the emotional center in the middle of our brain (Persinger et al., 2010). Basically, they attached emotional signals to the electromagnetic fields that were created by two helmets: the first one initially called the Koren helmet, but then named the God Helmet by a journalist, causing distress in the researchers; and the second one called the Octopus, which turned out to be better at facilitating telepathic experiences.

Telepathy in the Waking State

This Octopus helmet was the one used by Elizabeth Lloyd Mayer, the psychoanalyst who wrote the book *Extraordinary Knowing* (2007) about paranormal communication, which included Ullman and Krippner's telepathic dream studies and her visit to Persinger's lab many years later. She volunteered to participate in an experiment test for telepathic ability. All in all, she spent six hours at the lab, sitting in a comfortable chair inside an acoustic chamber, which greatly reduced the sound level. A student put the Octopus helmet over her head and ping-pong balls cut in half over her eyes. Inside the Octopus helmet were eight small solenoids, arranged in a circle, that created a very low-level electromagnetic field, lower than the field from a blow dryer, but greater than the earth's electromagnetic field, with emotional signals from the amygdala and the hippocampus embedded in the fields. The six hours passed quickly, and she was asked to say whatever came to her mind, something that felt comfortable to her, since that is an easy task for a psychoanalyst.

What she did not anticipate, though, was not knowing when she was in the telepathy experiment. She didn't know she had already participated until a student showed up with some colored postcards and asked her to rank them in order of how closely they corresponded to the images in her mind from the six hours of the experiments. She looked at all the cards, six of them, all very different: a merry-go-round, a bright sunset, an old-fashioned steam engine, and three scenes from the University campus. None of the images that she had seen corresponded to any of the cards. She told the graduate student she couldn't do it, meanwhile thinking to herself that she knew she was going to be a dead loss at telepathy. He insisted on reminding her that she had promised to come up with the rankings as part of her participation in the study. By now she really didn't care and knew the student just needed some data, so she glanced at the cards again and picked one. She picked the red sunset for the first one and went through the others at random. The student went to another room to get a sealed envelope with the target image; the postcard was the red sunset. Here is her description of how she felt:

> [A]t that moment, the world looked weird. I felt the tiniest instant of overwhelming fear. It was gone in a flash, but it was stunningly real. It was unlike any fear I've ever felt. My mind split. I realized that I knew something I was simultaneously certain I didn't know. And I got it. This is what my patients meant when they said, "My mind's not my own." Or "I'm losing my mind." The feeling was terrifying. My mind had slipped out from under me and the world felt out of control.
>
> (Mayer, 2007, p. 207)

When she was thinking about her experience later, she realized that she had come to the lab searching for words to label the feeling that came before she had felt the fear. The problem was she couldn't find words to name it. All the words were too definitive. The closest was to say she had felt "drawn" to the picture of the red sunset. But even that was too conclusive. It sounded as if she had been *conscious* of what she had done, but she hadn't been. She wasn't aware of any space between her and the picture of the sunset.

Her experience of fear about knowing something extraordinary, not through the usual five senses, is common for many people, but a number of other people are quite comfortable discovering that they have knowledge that seems telepathic. Richard Reichbart is one of those people. He is very used to having experiences of telepathic connection with his patients, and it goes both ways.

Like Reichbart, my patient is quite comfortable and even pleased to have this ability, although at first she said she does not want people to think she has "special powers." She is happy to have this special skill; she is aware that people might make fun of her or say she is deluded, so she has been very quiet about her ability, but overall, she values it as an unusual skill. It has helped her feel more powerful and aware of her own sense of agency, both with telepathic dreaming and with telepathic knowledge in the waking state, during our psychoanalytic work.

When the patient is comfortable with telepathic ability, her confidence increases and shifts the balance of power in the relationship with the analyst. This shift can have a good effect, as can anything that increases the power of the patient with respect to the analyst. Hoffman (2000) understands the power of this shift very well, although in his paper, he is talking about the effect of the analyst's old age and illness, not telepathic ability. His paper about his own patient's surprise visit in Hoffman's house after his heart atack is particularly poignant, as Hoffman describes his patient's reparative concern as Hoffman himself was struggling with his own mortality because of his life threatening situation. He goes on to say that in psychoanalytic work, "'progress' emerges as a kind of reparative gift, one that implicitly overcomes the patient's tendency to withhold such change out of a sense of chronic, malignant envy" (p. 823).

I had not thought about withholding progress because of envy in connection with my patient and our work together, but I believe that her telepathic gift definitely has made her feel more powerful and less resentful of aspects of me that do cause her to feel envious. One good effect of our discussions about her ability has been to increase cooperation with me in our work together by decreasing the envy. Experiencing my respect has made it much easier for her to gratify me both by making progress in our work together and in her life.

Psychoanalytic Research and the Level of Emotional Engagement

Psychoanalytic research has shown repeatedly that the therapeutic alliance, the strength of the relationship, which includes the level of emotional engagement, is the most important factor in getting a good treatment result. Unconscious communication has been more important than insight all along, since psychoanalysis began; however, Freud and other analysts took some time to figure it out. Since the beginning of psychoanalysis, Freud and other analysts have noticed extraordinary knowing, psi, and telepathy in the sessions, although only a few have reported them. Psychoanalysts and psychoanalytic therapists are now, once again, noticing how much the depth of the connections made in deep clinical work naturally overlap with telepathy.

The unconscious connection that makes psychotherapy and psychoanalysis an excellent place to study telepathy, both in dreams and in the waking state, is unrelated to the style of psychoanalysis. For example, telepathy has been reported no matter how talkative or quiet the analyst is during the treatment or whether the analyst is self-disclosing or abstinent. It is about a particular kind of unconscious communication that takes place between the analyst and analysand. They do not have to be in the same room. The work can take place on the phone or Zoom. Deep connections can take place across oceans; it is possible to have extraordinary knowledge from the other side of world.

Rupert Sheldrake and Morphic Resonance

Janine de Peyer (2016) describes the work of "leading yet controversial telepathy researcher" Rupert Sheldrake (1981, 2009, 2012; Sheldrake & Smart, 2003), whose theories of "morphic fields," "morphic resonance," and the "extended mind" were considered so provocative by the mainstream scientific community that his TED talk "The Science Delusion" (Sheldrake, 2013) was removed from distribution on TEDx YouTube's global Internet conferences. Sheldrake advocates that all human experiences and memories are stored in a nonlocal morphic field outside the brain, similar to the Hindu akashic records, a library containing all knowledge of human experience and the history of the cosmos, similar to Jung's collective unconscious. Sheldrake postulates a living, developing universe with its own memory. He views the mind as a field that extends beyond the physical brain, and the brain as receiver of information coming from a universal consciousness. Sheldrake views telepathy, which he considers a natural ability in animal groups, as innately possible among human beings. The human individual is seen as consciousness "honed in" from a greater morphic interconnectedness to compose a unique specificity or local mind. Sheldrake's morphic resonance is consistent with Persinger's research of electromagnetic fields, which is being continued by Todd Murphy (2019).

Telepathy in the Psychoanalytic Process in the Waking State

During a phone session within the last year, my patient's telepathic ability occurred in the waking state. Early in the session, I had noticed a very slight feeling on the left side of my neck and also around the middle of my neck—a tiny jolt. I felt unnerved. I had already experienced a difficulty using my left hand that I feared might be related to my neck. However, I immediately forgot about the tiny jolt until my patient said right in the middle of our session that she could feel the kind of shift that happens in her mind at times. This shift grabbed my attention because these shifts usually indicate an abrupt transition to a particular altered state of awareness, one which is obscure and still not well understood by either of us. This shift felt to her like an intrusion into what we were doing: We had begun some light hypnosis with an agreed upon intention to explore a particular issue on her mind, which she said was not urgent or especially important. (I use hypnosis in person, on Zoom, and on the phone, to induce light trance states when doing psychoanalysis with people who dissociate easily. I find it useful as an adjunct to our more free associative work, as it gives us better access to visual images.)

She reported a vague thought of something about a chicken—like a chicken wing; suddenly, she got an image of my neck. She then began expressing worries about my neck. At that point, I remembered the little jolt in my neck. My patient reported she was in an altered state of awareness, like a trance state, with gentle waves, kind of flowing. She was upset about the intrusion and thought, "Oh, come on—a chicken? What does that have to do with anything?" She said she tried to dismiss the thought and get her mind to "behave." Meanwhile, I had started to think about chickens' necks and was wondering what she was thinking about unconsciously about my neck. I began to think about a disturbing memory of a chicken I saw killed by wringing its neck. I wondered if some angry feelings were moving into working position in her unconscious and if she were having an unconscious idea about wringing a chicken's neck. It also occurred to me that idea was only a thought away from wringing my neck.

She then began talking to me about her worry about my neck, and my worries loomed again. She thought it was weird how it went from a chicken to a blur, and then to worry about my neck, and next to a chicken bone that might be like my neck. I then told her about my experience of feeling the jolt in my neck during our session, which I had forgotten about until she mentioned necks.

She said what a strange experience it was for her to be thinking about chicken necks and my neck, but she did not mention any aggressive thoughts. I believe she was not consciously aware of such thoughts about me at that time. It also did not occur to me that I, too, could be having unconscious aggressive thoughts about wringing necks—and yet remain consciously completely unaware of them. Not until I began working on this chapter did I begin to realize what might be going on in our unconsciouses, as part of our work on the negative transference and countertransference, which was ongoing.

My patient and I were having some kind of unusual communication that was different from our usual connection, and I began to realize it was likely that our minds were at similar levels of depth, similar altered states of awareness that were unconsciously created by both of us in the psychoanalytic work. This creation of unconscious communication was described very well by Isakower in the 1950s when he taught classes about the psychoanalytic instrument to candidates at the New York Psychoanalytic Institute.

The idea of the analytic instrument was first introduced by Freud around the idea of unconscious communication, then mentioned by Ferenczi in the *Clinical Diaries*. It operates silently, with one half in the analyst and the other in the patient. Isakower (Wyman & Rittenberg, 1992) has given the most complete description of it as he described his own experience:

> The analyzing instrument works unconsciously and, more than that, when it functions at its best, it is inaccessible to simultaneous observation, that is, conscious observation. It does not lend itself readily to being observed while operating. The characteristics of the analyzing instrument can be distinguished best in retrospect, when looking back at a portion of its work, a fraction of an individual session, not while it is doing the work, but immediately afterwards; most opportunely perhaps when that short phase of its intense functioning has occurred just before the end of an analytic session … Imagine with me, if you will, the end of one of your sessions. The session is broken off, the patient is leaving the room; you, the analyst, are in the process of emerging out of the "analytic situation"—that near dream-like state of hovering attention; the patient is being separated from you and you are left alone. In this short moment of the severance of the "team" you are left in midair and you become aware

> of the denuded raw surface of your half of the analyzing instrument, the surface which is opposite the patient's half.
>
> (p. 202)

My patient and I were experiencing a particular altered state of awareness that operated like the psychoanalytic instrument and, in addition, included a telepathic communication. It was similar to what Michael Balint (1955) reports in his paper on parapsychology and parapsychological healing:

> Quite gradually it then dawned upon me that in all cases of this kind there was a particular emotional situation between the analyst and his patient. As the situation was not quite unexceptionable, and moreover it was always my fault that it had arisen, I felt rather ashamed and reluctant to publish my mistakes in print.
>
> Briefly, the situation can be described as highly ambivalent and extremely tense … Usually, the patient was in a state of intense positive dependent transference, which however was not fully appreciated and understood by the analyst. The cause of this lack of appreciation and understanding was without exception some transitory preoccupation on the analyst's part, which at the material time absorbed a greater part of his attention than was good for the progress of the analysis. The patient in his helpless dependence reacted to this by renewed efforts to win the analyst's full attention, and in this very tense situation, bordering on despair, an apparently telepathic and clairvoyant phenomenon occurred. The result was always a surprise, almost a shock, to the analyst, and had the effect of bringing him round, as he could not help giving more attention than in the immediately preceding period to a patient who was producing such highly interesting and puzzling phenomena. In this way the very tense ambivalent situation resolved itself and the analysis resumed its normal course.
>
> (p. 32)

Later in the same paper, Balint writes,

> Against the realization that in the production of apparent E.S.P. phenomena the analyst's ambivalent counter-transference has a large share, the two defensive mechanisms … are mobilized: projection (it is the patient who produces the E.S.P. phenomena) and idealization (E.S.P. is a highly interesting scientific problem—and is not emotional, is not caused by suffering).
>
> (p. 33)

I realized that I could be having unconscious aggressive thoughts about my patient as part of our ongoing work on her understandable disappointment and resentment; the aggression was not just being communicated by her. Balint's experience of not giving the patient full attention applies to me, since I was preoccupied with my left hand and a worry that it was caused by something wrong in my neck. I was not giving my full attention to my patient and her dependency needs—or any needs she had at that time. Her startling ideas about the chicken and then the necks got my immediate attention, however, and at first, I thought she was the one producing the phenomenon. However, I later understood that both of us were at similar levels of depth and preoccupied with aggression.

Who started this unconscious communication, and when? How did it happen? An important part was her strong need to connect with me and to have my full attention that resonated with her deep disappointment and resentment about her unmet dependency needs in childhood and throughout her life. The telepathic communication emerged from our unconscious psychoanalytic process as part of our ongoing work on these negative feelings. My lapse of attention contributed to the unconscious process that was created by both of us, so no one is totally responsible, although the responsibility for creating a therapeutic analytic process without aggression or retaliation is assigned to the analyst, as part of the privileged position of having greater knowledge. However, our unconscious communication was part of a necessary psychoanalytic process to address these issues, a process that was shaped by two imperfect human beings. Nonetheless, I agree with Balint that it is embarrassing to acknowledge aggressive countertransferential issues. Moreover, as Balint points out, analysts and therapists have been prone to see telepathy as posing a very interesting scientific problem and have avoided acknowledging some of the painful emotion that is embedded in the communication. During the work with my patient, I have become more aware of how much suffering and strong emotion are a part of telepathic communication. The need for connection and inclusion to alleviate feelings of loss and being left out are very important, as Eshel (this volume) understands very well.

Conclusion

In this chapter, I have provided two examples of what I believe to be telepathic communications—one from a dream and one from the waking state. The dream about my new home office occurred 14 years before the experience of her conscious communication of telepathic knowledge about my neck in the waking state. Our talking about the dream from time to time in our work seems to have deepened the psychoanalytic process more than I expected. Our discussions about the dream have been extremely important for me and have helped me focus more on inchoate and evanescent feeling states in my countertransference, and I am more aware of different aspects of her personality. Her startling knowledge about my neck that occurred recently in the waking state is probably only a small part of our ongoing unconscious communication, some of it telepathic, and not consciously experienced by either of us.

For both of us, acknowledging telepathy has been very important for our work together, and my being able to show her the lake and the porch, and how correct she was, when she came to my new office, communicated my respect for her ability. Our repeated discussions of the dream have also been very important for her increasing cooperation with me, making it easier for her to make steady progress in her understanding of herself and in her life. We both have felt gratified by being able to participate in this experience.

References

Balint, M. (1955). Notes on parapsychology and parapsychological healing. *International Journal of Psychoanalysis*, 36, 31–35.

de Peyer, J. (2016). Uncanny communication and the porous mind. *Psychoanalytic Dialogues*, 26, 156–174.

Ferenczi, S. (1932/1988). *The clinical diary of Sándor Ferenczi* (J. Dupont, Ed.; M. Balint & N. Z. Jackson, Trans.). Harvard University Press.

Freud, S.(1953). A discovery like that comes only once in a lifetime. Introduction to *The interpretation of dreams*, 4 (J. Strachey, Ed.; p. xx). (Original work published in 1899.)

Hoffman, I. Z. (2000). At death's door: Therapists and patients as agents. *Psychoanalytic Dialogues*, 10, 821–846.

Mayer, E. L. (2007). *Extraordinary knowing*. Bantam.

Murphy, T. (2019). Solving the "hard problem": Consciousness as an intrinsic property of magnetic fields. *Journal of Consciousness Exploration & Research*, 10, 646–659.

Persinger, M. A., Saroka, K. S., Koren, S. A., & St-Pierre, L. S. (2010). The electromagnetic induction of mystical and altered states within the laboratory. *Journal of Consciousness Exploration & Research*, 1, 808–830.

Reichbart, R. (2019). *The paranormal surrounds us: Psychic phenomena in literature, culture and psychoanalysis.* McFarland.

Sheldrake, R. (1981). *A new science of life: A hypothesis of formative causation*. J. P. Tarcher.

Sheldrake, R. (2009). *Morphic resonance: The nature of formative causation*. Park Street Press.

Sheldrake, R. (2012). *The science delusion: Freeing the spirit of enquiry*. Coronet.

Sheldrake, R. (2013). TEDx Whitechapel. Retrieved from www.sheldrake.org/videos/the-science-delusion.

Sheldrake, R., & Smart, P. (2003). Experimental tests for telephone telepathy. *Journal of the Society for Psychical Research*, 67, 184–199.

Wyman, H. M. & Rittenberg, S. M. (Eds.) (1992). The analyzing instrument in the teaching and conduct of the analytic process of Otto Isakower, M.D.. *Journal of Clinical Psychoanalysis*, 1, 200–203.

Chapter 11

Thinking of Mystics and Mysticism with Bion

João Carlos Braga

This chapter introduces the work of João Braga, MD, a prominent Brazilian analyst, whom we are fortunate to have joining us. João is a Bionian and expounds here on Bionion theory. After presenting two telepathic communications from patients (one having to do with a patient telepathically and unconsciously intuiting the sudden appearance of a supervisor of his analyst, and the other having to do with a patient telepathically dreaming of a birthday party for João's nine-year-old grandson). João indicates how telepathy must be related to the primordial mind that Bion posits and states how telepathy develops "a deep interconnection between analyst and analysand (being at one with 'O') [and] moves the psychoanalytic boundaries into the unknown."

* * * *

Bion's late contributions to psychoanalysis (1970–79) sparked a growing clinical interest in observing experiences of intense emotional interconnection between analyst and analysand (*being at one*). This shift offers an opportunity for discussions about the boundaries between psychoanalytic knowledge and events traditionally attributed to supernatural powers by laymen. For psychoanalysts, this intense emotional involvement of analyst/analysand fosters the analysand's experience with their own mental functioning and reveals itself as an opportunity to investigate the enigmatic psychic realm of mystics as part of our natural primitive mental functioning. The belief in such phenomena spans a group of manifestations, such as telepathy, telepathic dreams, thought-transference, premonitions, mediumship, divination, and peculiar bodily manifestations. These manifestations possibly represent the surface of a vast domain. Although they lack a consistent psychological understanding, they prompt us to contemplate them within the framework of the natural mental world.

The psychoanalytic stance toward these fringe territories can be traced back to Freud's scientific curiosity, which revolutionized the study of the human mind. Despite facing scrutiny, Freud (1921, 1922, 1925, 1933) ventured into exploring the phenomena of telepathy and thought-transference, but he temporarily set them aside to safeguard psychoanalysis from accusations of mysticism. Eighty

DOI: 10.4324/9781003611042-12

years later, psychoanalytic knowledge significantly evolved beyond its initial scope, delving into new areas like psychotic functioning, the primitive mind (M. Klein), the ontological dimensions of the psyche (Bion and Winnicott), and the primordial mind (Bion), extending the scientific boundaries into the unknown.

Based on Bion's proposals, a psychoanalytic approach to these transcendent manifestations would depend on the analyst enabling direct engagement with undifferentiated elements evolving from psychic reality (Bion, 1965). This access requires Faith (F) in the existence of a non-sensuous psychic reality (Bion, 1970). With this stance, psychoanalytic interests superpose dimensions typically relevant to religion, occultism, and lay mysticism.

Before discussing Bion's ideas conceptually, I would like to include some clinical material on this topic as an introduction.

Clinical Experiences: Two Telepathic Dreams

Within the consulting room, analysts witness a broad spectrum of experiences within themselves, their patients, and the analytic relationship. The quality of these observations depends on the analysts' own psychoanalytic development; experiences beyond their expertise may register as mere cognitive data, lacking integration into the psychoanalyst's personality. If the analyst is receptive to transcendent experiences, observations may acquire germinal meanings revealing crucial mental processes striving for consciousness and integration.

So-called paranormal phenomena are frequently treated by laypersons as having a metaphysical origin, generating a belief in supernatural powers. For psychoanalysts, the discussion of these phenomena is essential to open their eyes to the existence of manifestations of a mysterious mental dimension, endowing them to experience and investigate these natural events. Also, the presence of these phenomena opens a rich opportunity to help analysands to give birth to parts of their personality. So, even if paranormal phenomena lack consistent psychological explanations, it is possible to look at them as pertaining to the natural mental world and think of them as manifestations of what Freud named unconscious.

Some of these experiences have a profound impact on the analyst and generate a conviction in their natural existence. Telepathic dreams are perhaps the most convincing experience of this kind, and I will use them to illustrate our incursion as psychoanalysts in this realm, which we share with mystics and mysticism.

A Vignette with a Telepathic Dream[1]

An analysand, Herbert, experienced a dream in which he intuited that his analyst had started supervision of his analysis. It emerged during an online session:

HERBERT: I had a peculiar dream. It was my first dream involving you. We were in a session, both in person and online simultaneously. There was a man, Ricardo Amorim,[2] lying on your bed. Do you know him?

ANALYST: The dream is all yours.

HERBERT: [chuckling before continuing] In the dream, a guy was in the middle of our session. He directed questions through you, but you seemed clueless as you relayed them to me. Meanwhile, by my side, there was a young woman, a famous actress, scantily clad, urging me to abandon our session. Quite an entourage, don't you think? Oh, and do you happen to know Ricardo Amorim?

ANALYST: Your dream seems to convey something significant. What do you think it says about our relationship, our dynamic as analyst and analysand?

HERBERT: Indeed, I wonder if, once we return to in-person sessions, I can hug you. It's been so long since we've seen each other.

ANALYST: [caught off guard] I already feel hugged. [The air seemed to momentarily stand still.]

HERBERT: We can discuss that later, alright?

ANALYST: I'm getting the idea that you never lived a relationship like ours—a connection characterized by profound psychic intimacy yet devoid of physical touch.

HERBERT: Yes, it's a unique dynamic for me to navigate.

A Session with a Telepathic Dream[3]

Stan arrives at the session visibly tense. He was about to undergo a prostate biopsy for a suspicious image detected on ultrasound, a finding that he had talked about during previous sessions. Stan talks in detail about the biopsy and his ideas about it. He extends his observations to memories surrounding his father's death due to the same disease, which, even before undergoing the biopsy, Stan already believed that he had. He highlights the fact that his current age is the same as his father's when he died.

While listening to him, I feel increasingly uncomfortable. That session would be the last one before my summer vacation, and I started to consider postponing my trip to avoid leaving him alone at that difficult moment. These feelings and thoughts make me aware of the presence of guilt.

The emotional atmosphere in the session is intense and has hints of terror. Suddenly, Stan mentions bluntly: "I thought I wouldn't tell you, but I've already decided that if the biopsy shows cancer, I won't come back for the sessions." His surprising comment makes me more uncomfortable, followed by his silence, as if he were waiting for my response. After a tense moment, I said to him: "We don't know what the biopsy will show, but we can both already follow that you are having doubts about our condition of dealing together with a situation that is very scary for you." My words seem to wake him to my presence, and he begins to include me in his associations. He points out two or three situations in which he recognizes the analysis as playing an essential role in his life. He surprised me by describing a dream, which he rarely did in his sessions. In his dream, he arrives at one of his sessions, and the door to the consultation room is closed. While in the waiting room, he somehow knew that I was in session with a boy, and because of that, I would not call him in. He also realizes in the dream that a party was going on in another part of the house, to which he was not invited. After describing this dream, he makes no associations but casually adds that the boy was nine years old.

After describing the dream, Stan remains silent. His description makes me feel profoundly disturbed and perplexed because, the next day, I was traveling on vacation to meet with family members and celebrate my nine-year-old grandson's birthday, something that had been strongly present in my mind. I will make a brief assessment of the situation, but I am unable to identify possible sources from which Stan could have known this information about my personal life. I feel compelled to intervene but, simultaneously, unsure about what path to take. My first thought was to follow the path of symbolic formation and propose that he was the boy—and not the adult—who primarily needed my care. However, my emotional experience weighs on me. After some hesitation and struggle with my fears, I tell him: "It seems to me that you have a knowledge not known to you, the knowledge that there is a boy with whom I will be with when I leave you at this challenging time for you." A heavy, prolonged silence follows, as if we had lost the ground on which we stood. Stan looks very surprised by my unusual statement, and I am amazed at the experience that I was living. The atmosphere in the session becomes awkward, disturbing, and overwhelming, but the tension eases gradually. As the session continues, a layer of deep intimacy emerges between us. His communications flow easily, allowing us to look at the ongoing emotional situation from various vertices. Stan communicates his belief that he is facing an imminent disaster and revives, with lively emotion, memories of situations that we have already analyzed. He brings up rivalries that he had with his younger sister since childhood, delusional beliefs about a predetermined fate of a cancer death following his family history, and the fact that he had to be resigned to subordinate positions in affective relationships based on his certainty that his father had always preferred his sister to him. Stan appeared to be self-analyzing in my presence, and my participation in the remaining session became limited to punctual interventions and expansions (approximations and integrations) of his elaborations. For example, I told him what he was doing in my company was like revising a poorly elaborated draft.

Bion's Contributions

Bion proposed three seminal shifts to the traditional psychoanalytic understanding of the mind: (1) a transition from a biological (drives) to a psychological (thinking) standpoint (1961–65); (2) a focus shift from an epistemological view ("what is represented") to an ontological one ("what is unknown and even unknowable") (1965–70); (3) the inclusion of psychoanalytical attention to the existence of an inaccessible prenatal mind (1976–79), beyond the dimensions of conscious and unconscious. For our current exploration of the nature of mysticism, mystics, telepathy, and thought-transference, it is worth emphasizing the latter two of these contributions.

Would "Being at One" Be the Base for Thought-Transference?

In *Transformations* (1965), Bion proposed the theory of transformations in being or becoming reality ("O"). He later developed further these ideas in *Attention and Interpretation* (1970). In both books, Bion proposes the identification and operationality of the human capacity for direct approach to psychic reality. This theory points out the expansion of the boundaries of psychoanalysis beyond its traditional realm of knowing and not knowing, ushering psychoanalysis into a new psychic domain. Bion termed this new domain "O" (from Origin), denoting the ultimate, unknowable essence of things—whether material or immaterial. Accessing this realm of the unknowable—which is inaccessible to knowledge but accessible to experience—requires faith ("F") in its existence and in its potential to experience and utilize elements of the undifferentiated layer of the mind. With it, Bion endeavored to establish a disciplined psychoanalytical approach for engaging the level of undifferentiated psychic functioning, that is out of human understanding.

Bion's efforts happened within a scientific framework. This approach opens a window to investigate these transcendent events treated as supernormal. This scientific approach to events moves us closer to manifestations of two minds somehow sharing the same experience without sensorial stimuli.

The conjecture herein is that this experience of deep interconnection between analyst and analysand is the base for the occurrence of intuition, thought transference, and telepathy. With Bion, intuition emerged as the most crucial psychoanalytic tool for apprehending the constant conjunctions arising from the non-symbolic dimension. It is essential to discern that this intuition does not entail grasping the unknowable thing-in-itself, but rather encompasses knowledge derived from lived experiences.

From my clinical experience, two authors have significantly expanded upon Bion's ideas in this topic. One is Ofra Eshel (2006, 2019a, 2019b), through her clinical and theoretical inquiries into states of deep interconnection between analyst and analysand, bridging the gap between knowledge and being, as posited by Bion (1965). Also, Eshel's clinical investigations on treating archaic mental states and her studies on telepathic phenomena significantly contribute to this topic. The other author is Andre Green (1998), who introduced the concept of postnatal not yet born thoughts as part of the domain of the primordial mind, in association with Bion's conjectures on prenatal proto-thoughts and proto-feelings.

Is Primordial Mind the Base for Extrasensory Perception?

In his last three years of life (1976–79), Bion frequently referenced the presence of vestiges of a prenatal mind in grown-up persons. He has done that in papers, seminars, and supervisions but has not organized them theoretically. In his Seminars in Los Angeles (1976), New York (1977), Rome (1977), and São Paulo (1978), Bion made rich references to the existence of this primary layer of the mind before birth and the establishment of object relationships. He named it the *inaccessible*:

> If, as I suggested before, the embryo tries to get rid itself of unpleasant and unwelcome primordial sensations, it could have "ideas" or "feelings" that *never had at any time been conscious*. The nearest I can get to describing it is that these "ideas" or "feelings" where "available" or "not available": they have become out of reach of their Origin. So, when you are dealing with a grown person you will have to distinguish between something conscious or unconscious and something inaccessible.
>
> (Bion, 1978, p. 105)

Two intertwined points interest us for our present topic. First, the embryological knowledge that the central nervous system of the embryo and fetus is the thalamus, since the brain cortex has not developed yet. Second, the conjecture that there are embryonic primitive sensors in this phase that our postnatal sensorial development covers. These conjectures permit us to wonder if telepathy and thought-transference have their roots in the existence of primordial sensors capable of receiving impressions and registering them in the thalamus-adrenals axis, that will develop as the autonomic nervous system in the postnatal mind.

Bion's Ideas on Mysticism and Mystics

Vermote (2019) synthesizes the relationship between psychoanalysts and mysticism as seen by Bion:

> Mysticism adopts a different approach than philosophy by saying that one cannot know O but one has to become it. For the mystic, the direct contact with an Ultimate Reality is a life-changing experience, for which there are no words; it is an experience that can only be addressed indirectly. This experience is described as an illumination or satori in Zen. Bion does not advocate such a mystic experience, but he focuses on the getting to know, the experience of the unknowable emotional essence of a psychoanalytic session.
>
> (p. 127)

In other words, mystic experiences are not supernatural but a mental predisposition that creates a receptivity to undifferentiated elements that naturally evolve from their Origin ("O"), the psychic reality. Analysts, like Freud, inevitably believe in a reality that exists in the depth of our psyches.

There are at least three moments in Bion's work where he is explicit in his thinking about mystics and mysticism. Let us dive deeper into each one of them.

We can wonder whether, in Chapter 6 of *Attention and Interpretation* ("The Mystic and the Group"), Bion (1970) was answering the criticism that he was adopting a mystic vision of mental life when proposing a transcendent view of the mind with his ideas on transformations in being or becoming reality. Bion directly tackled this theme when he dared to use the expression "act of faith" to refer to a scientific faith in the existence of things that:

> cannot be known by any human being; it can be known about, its presence can be recognized and felt, but it cannot be known. It is possible to be at one with it. That it exists is an essential postulate of science but it cannot be scientifically discovered.
>
> (p. 30)

Some pages beyond, Bion points out the primary characteristics of mystics:

> From this conviction of inaccessibility of absolute reality, the mystics must be exempted. Their inability to express themselves through the medium of ordinary language, art or music is related to the fact that all such methods of communication are transformations and transformations deals with phenomena and are dealt with by being known, loved or hated—K, L or H.
>
> (p. 147)

In the Italian seminars, Bion touched twice on ideas within the borders between psychoanalytic established knowledge and mysticism. In the sixth seminar, Bion elaborated on a question by one participating analyst, who described his experience with an analysand who reported a dream with events very similar to those he (the analyst) had painfully lived just hours before. Bion answered cautiously but positively about the existence in humans of other senses beyond the ones that we recognize, as well as of the sixth sense (consciousness) that Freud described as the sensory organ for psychic quality, and of the seventh that he (Bion) had conceptualized as intuition in *Attention and Interpretation* (1970). In the Italian seminar, Bion (1977) states: "But the questions that have been raised here may mean that we have to become aware of the possibility that there are other receptor organs of which we are not aware" (p. 64).

This same conjecture of the possible existence of "other senses" can also be found a few pages before the above quotation. Bion recalls a clinical experience with a very disturbed patient with a dramatic beginning of a life. He states: "to draw the patients' attention to vestiges of acute observation—so acute that they could not stand the information that their primordial senses brought them" (p. 52).

We find another conjecture by Bion (1978) on this theme in the fourth seminar in New York:[4]

> There are certain things which we would nowadays call thoughts or ideas but which are really physical. I am dubious about using terms like "the adrenals" and "the optic thalamus" when I am talking about the mind. I shall never know whether there is any such thing or not, but I think it is convenient to leave one or two boxes empty in case somebody is able to fill them up.
>
> (p. 49)

A broader description of the presence of these primary sensors is present in *Cogitations* (1992), a transcript from a tape recording from August 8, 1978. In it, Bion sets the biological base for phenomena that are out of reach of our everyday senses and logical thinking. We can extend it, at least as a conjecture, to paranormal phenomena:

> These poets and artists have their methods of recording their awareness of some sort of influence, stimuli that come from without, the unknown that is so terrifying, such a powerful feeling that they cannot be described in ordinary terms. They have to be considered to be perceivable only in so far as the human being has thalamic organs and thalamic experiences, and as if the human mind itself, described in physical terms, were a central nervous system that has only developed as far as the thalamus, thus leaving no real synaptic communication between the thalamus and the subsequent development of the mind, the neopalliun, or whatever the appropriate term for it should be. We need to invent some form of articulate speech that could approximate to describing these realities, the phenomena that I cannot possibly describe.
>
> (p. 369)

Wrapping Ip

This chapter prioritizes two topics drawn from Bion's insights into the undeveloped mind. First, it addresses the evolution of his theory on the profound interconnectedness between analyst and analysand, leading to transformative shifts in the apprehension of reality through intuition—the mental function that could base telepathy. Second, it approaches Bion's speculations on the existence of primordial sensors in grown-up people, remnants of a prenatal proto mind. Both these topics represent novel psychoanalytic perspectives on the enigmatic realm of unconscious communication, opening new vertices for theoretical exploration and clinical practice.

The analysand's telepathic dreams described above bring attention to a central point of this topic: For decades, different authors collected psychoanalytical evidence that somehow experiences of one mind are caught and dreamt by another mind without sensorial communication. This experience converges with Freud's proposal of unconscious communication and Bion's (1977) proposal that we are glimpsing at yet another dimension of the mind, beyond conscious and unconscious, the *inaccessible* one.

We don't have conclusive positions from Bion on *mysticism*, but we do have strong stances on the subject *mystic*. In Vermote's (2019) summary, we find a brief encapsulation of this notion:

> To Bion, adopting this instance is not a mystical experience in itself; he is not looking for a state of bliss. Bion's aim is not mystical enlightenment but a psychic change within the well-defined psychoanalytic frame, which is different from a religious experience.
>
> (p. 150)

Later,

> One could also argue that he made a rational progression in his thinking, leading him to use mystical metaphors in theory and practice in his transcendental period without really realizing them from within as mystics do. Ultimately, he transformed them in a more philosophical Socratic stance of fundamental not-knowing in thinking about psychoanalysis in his lectures and supervisions of this last period.
>
> (p. 233)

The speculation here is that developing a deep interconnection between analyst and analysand (*being at one with "O"*) moves the psychoanalytic boundaries into the unknown. The previously conquered boundaries, including intuition and at-one-ment in the psychoanalytic domains, already have created a common ground for many analysts to investigate telepathic phenomena. Bion's epistemological position on these proposals is essential for approaching the topic. This chapter highlights his theories to explain these phenomena and its existence: "I don't think my explanation matters. What I would draw attention to is the *nature* of the problem" (Bion, 1978, p. 107).

My understanding of Bion's position is that he chooses a standpoint that privileges *what* is happening and not *why* it is happening, that is, the facts that different persons with different backgrounds can recognize—and not the interpretation they give to them. This understanding brings us to two central ideas in the knowledge of mystic manifestations: On a psychological level, there is the human capacity to create a common area between two minds in which mysterious phenomena happen; on a biological level, we carry within ourselves remnants of our prenatal development, with primordial sensors to psychic events that are capable of capturing non-sensuous feelings in a way that our ordinary sensorial senses do not do.

In accordance with these ideas, Bion advocated that mystics are exceptional individuals ("geniuses"), fundamental to the development of any group for their capacity to "see" elements of the undifferentiated dimension of the mind. This dimension pre-exists the development of knowledge: "I shall use the term 'mystic' to describe these exceptional individuals. I include scientists, and Newton is the outstanding example of such a man" (Bion, 1970, p. 64).

Within this meaning, we are confronted with a puzzling conclusion: Bion could be classified as a mystic—a scientific mystic—as would be Freud, Melanie Klein, and every analyst who develops the conviction that it is rewarding in psychoanalysis to approach the undifferentiated layer of the mind.

Notes

1 My thanks to Luciane Fioravante Morais for letting me use this vignette.
2 Ricardo Amorim is a well-known Brazilian economist.
3 Clinical material presented by the author in the paper "The Oneiric Dimensions of the Mind" at Bion's International Conference, Mexico City, 2022.
4 Curiously, these 1977 New York Seminars were promoted by IPTAR (Institute for Psychoanalytic Training and Research), the same institution that organized the meeting on which this chapter is based.

References

Bion, W. R. (1965). *Transformations.* Karnac.

Bion, W. R. (1970). *Attention and interpretation.* Karnac.

Bion, W. R. (1977). *Taming wild thoughts* (F. Bion, Ed.). Karnac.

Bion, W. R. (1978). *Bion in New York and São Paulo.* Clunie Press.

Bion, W. R. (1992). *Cogitations* (F. Bion, Ed.). Karnac.

Eshel, O. (2006). Where are you, my beloved? *International Journal of Psychoanalysis*, 87, 1603–1627.

Eshel, O. (2019a). Would clinical psychoanalysis shy away from delving further into the unknown? On the mystery of telepathic dreams. *International Journal of Psychoanalysis*, 100, 608–610.

Eshel, O. (2019b). *The emergence of analytic oneness: Into the heart of psychoanalysis.* Routledge.

Freud, S. (1921). Psychoanalysis and telepathy. In J. Strachey (Ed. & Trans.), *The standard edition of the complete psychological works of Sigmund Freud* (Vol. 18, pp. 177–193). Hogarth Press.

Freud, S. (1922). Dreams and telepathy. In J. Strachey (Ed. & Trans.), *The standard edition of the complete psychological works of Sigmund Freud* (Vol. 18, pp. 197–220). Hogarth Press.

Freud, S. (1925). Some additional notes upon dream interpretation. In J. Strachey (Ed. & Trans.), *The standard edition of the complete psychological works of Sigmund Freud* (Vol. 19, pp. 123–138). Hogarth Press.

Freud, S. (1933). Dreams and occultism. In J. Strachey (Ed. & Trans.), *The standard edition of the complete psychological works of Sigmund Freud* (Vol. 22, pp. 31–55). Hogarth Press.

Green, A. (1998). The primordial mind and the work of the negative. *International Journal of Psychoanalysis*, 79, 649–665.

Vermote, R. (2019). *Reading Bion*. Routledge.

Chapter 12

Psychoanalysis and Magic

Then and Now[1]

Mikita Brottman

Mikita Brottman, Ph.D., psychoanalyst and author of Phantoms of the Clinic: From Thought Transference to Projective Identification *(Karnac, 2011) is from Maryland, and here considers the long-standing and complex association between psychoanalysis and the paranormal. Beginning with a brief discussion of the early history of the psychoanalytic movement, she then takes up the subject of the paranormal in relation to the earliest practitioners of psychoanalysis, including Freud. Although magic, symbol, and superstition are generally considered to be primitive forms of thinking, contemporary psychoanalysis is full of them. She suggests that the tools of psychoanalysis can reveal some fascinating aspects of the modern human condition by showing how deeply we rely on primitive impulses. At the end of the chapter, Mikita examines how the connections between psychoanalysis and the paranormal have been extended and developed over time, with particular emphasis on the work of the psychiatrist, psychoanalyst, and paranormal investigator Jule Eisenbud.*

* * * *

> If I had to live my life over again, I should devote myself to psychical research, rather than psychoanalysis.
>
> Sigmund Freud, letter to Hereward Carrington (1921)
> (Jones, 1957, p. 392)

I

The rapid spread of spiritualism in Europe and America in the 1850s and 1860s quickly led to the rise of rationalist circles devoted to exploring the unexplained phenomena apparently produced by trances and séances. In Britain, one of these circles became the Society for Psychical Research, which was established in 1882 when a number of spiritualists and Cambridge scholars grew determined to place their belief in psychic phenomena upon a sound, unprejudiced footing grounded in the "scientific method." A new model of the unconscious mind emerged in the many publications of this

DOI: 10.4324/9781003611042-13

society's members (see Koutstaal, 1992; Noll, 1997; Shamdasani, 1993;), who considered such phenomena as trance states, crystal gazing, and automatic writing to be perfectly valid psychological methods for studying what they referred to as the "subliminal self." Indeed, Léon Chertok and Raymond de Saussure, in *The Therapeutic Revolution* (1973), draw a connection between the Victorian obsession with psychic phenomena and the "new science" of psychoanalysis—in particular, the Freudian concept of transference. The connection, according to Chertok and de Saussure, goes back to August 1885, when Freud first began studying hypnotism under the auspices of Jean-Martin Charcot at the Salpêtrière hospital in Paris. Freud's interest in the subject reflected the widespread public fascination with mysterious states of mind, including somnambulism, magnetism, catalepsy, nervous illness, and the fragmentation of personality. His later speculations about the unconscious mind were deeply influenced by the work of Charcot, especially his use of hypnosis to relieve the various automatic phenomena induced by hysteria.

Throughout his life, Freud never lost this fascination with unconscious (but active) ideas, and, at least in his younger days, often acknowledged the connections between psychoanalysis and magic. The following passage, from his 1890 essay "Psychical (or Mental) Treatment" (written when he was 34), provides a neat summary of his position at this time:

> A layman will no doubt find it hard to understand how pathological disorders of the body and mind can be eliminated by "mere" words. He will feel that he is being asked to believe in magic. And he will not be so very wrong, for the words which we use in our everyday speech are nothing other than watered down magic. But we shall have to follow a roundabout path in order to explain how science sets about restoring to words at least a part of their former magical power.
>
> (p. 285)

Quite clearly, anyone who expresses a belief in magic lays him- or herself open to accusations of credulity, but Freud was careful to emphasize that he was not in the least bit superstitious. In *The Psychopathology of Everyday Life* (1901), he wrote: "I believe in external (real) chance, it is true, but not in internal (psychical) accidental events. With superstitious persons it is the other way round" (p. 257).

By 1918, Freud was no longer writing full-blown case studies, and his work, though interesting in other ways, never resumed the intriguing, mysterious tone it achieves in his earlier works such as *Studies in Hysteria* (Breuer & Freud, 1895), where he and Breuer seem more like alchemists or Svengalis than a pair of respectable physicians. One might even say that, before the publication of *Studies in Hysteria*, Freud was more mesmerist than medic. According to Peter J. Swales (1986), Freud was known as *der Zauberer* ("the Magician") by the children of Anna von Lieben, a rich patient whom he treated at home in the 1880s. Not quite a "proper doctor," he was, claims Swales, generally received at the back door of his patients' homes, rather than the front. It does not seem surprising, then, that in his early work, Freud cast himself as a magician of the word.

In his later years, in fact, Freud expressed regret that he had not devoted himself more seriously to paranormal investigation. Ernest Jones (1957), in his biography, quotes the passage from a letter Freud wrote in 1921 to the British spiritualist and psychic researcher Hereward Carrington, which I have taken as the epigraph to this chapter. This avowal, with its "rather than" construction, suggests that, as Freud grew older and his work became increasingly well respected, he began to realize that the two fields of study—psychoanalysis and psychical research—were mutually exclusive, a position that solidified later in his career, when he expressed ambivalence about whether or not to continue his investigations into thought-transference.

When Freud first began his research, the field of psychiatry was rapidly disentangling itself from the realm of the spiritual. His main concern was that, if people began to associate psychoanalysis with the occult and supernatural, its reputation might be seriously endangered. His doubts were fostered and encouraged by Jones, who was openly embarrassed by Freud's interest in the occult and who persuaded him to forge closer affiliations between his "new science" and medicine, connections which, Jones felt, would considerably enhance the respectability and prestige of psychoanalysis. "We are physicians, and wish to remain physicians," Freud told Otto Gross at the 1908 Salzburg psychoanalytic conference when Gross spoke on "the cultural perspectives of science" (Schwentker, 1987, p. 488). Not long after this, however, psychoanalytic authors began publishing articles on European culture as a whole—its myths, fairy tales, literature, opera, and so on, attracting the attention of many readers and thinkers in fields far beyond that of science.

For his own part, Freud was anxious that his ideas about thought-transference might be misunderstood and possibly appropriated by spiritualists and mystics eager to prove that the universe contains more than material forms. Consequently, during the writing of *Totem and Taboo* (1913), he clashed famously with Jung, struggling to resist the seductive mysticism of his close friend and colleague's work. When *Totem and Taboo* was finally published, Jung was dismayed to discover that Freud came down stoutly in favor of a material, mechanistic theory of scientific rationalism. In his autobiographical work *Memories, Dreams, Reflections* (1961), Jung observed that Freud's fear of the occult sometimes verged on the histrionic, and it does not seem outlandish to speculate that, for Freud, supernatural manifestations resonated with a particular significance. In defense, Freud began to rationalize spiritual belief as a form of primitive thinking typical of children and psychotics, which, in *Totem and Taboo*, he refers to as "animism." According to Freud (1913), "primitive races … people the world with innumerable spiritual beings both benevolent and malignant; and these spirits and demons they regard as the causes of natural phenomena" (p. 76).

Although, in public, Freud worked hard to keep the boundaries of psychoanalysis distinct from those of the occult, in private, as Jones (1957) describes in his biography, Freud exhibited "an exquisite oscillation between skepticism and credulity" (p. 375) on the subject. Not only did he express constant anxiety about the assimilation of psychoanalysis into the realm of science, he often expressed his belief that the occult was inextricable from psychoanalysis, which, he believed, in order to be effective, had to embrace those manifestations of thought and emotion that are normally excluded from rational, scientific study. And while he remained ambivalent and conflicted about the more otherworldly reaches of occult belief, he always considered thought-transference to be the most respectable element in occultism, and the main "kernel of truth in the field" (Freud, 1922, p. 136). In fact, he believed the phenomenon would soon be incorporated into the realm of scientific fact. In "A Note on the Unconscious in Psychoanalysis" (1912), published in the *Proceedings of the Society for Psychical Research*, he wrote that, as far as he was concerned, future evidence from analysts would soon "put an end to any remaining doubts on the reality of thought-transference" (p. 266).

The late 1940s and early 1950s saw a resurgence of interest in the subject of the paranormal in the field of psychoanalysis, with numerous publications by Jule Eisenbud, Jan Ehrenwald, Nandor Fodor, and other notable scholar-practitioners. Today, psychoanalytic thinkers with an interest in such topics generally gravitate toward the field of transpersonal psychology, which deals with areas beyond rational ego-functioning, such as consciousness studies, near-death experiences, spiritual inquiry, body–mind relationships, and personal transformation. In transpersonal therapy or analysis, mystical experiences are often regarded as a form of "regression in the service of the ego," to use the term attributable to Ernst Kris (1952). Such experiences are generally believed to provide meaningful moments in the process of a human life. In other words, the transpersonal school entertains the possibility that at least some kinds of mystical experiences may be genuinely numinous.

In transpersonal therapy, patients generally work on developing their self-awareness beyond the limits of the body and the personal realm of experience. In earlier days, this kind of therapy was sometimes enhanced by the use of LSD and other psychedelics, but today's practitioners generally limit themselves to less controversial methods, such as breathwork or re-birthing. The field is currently gaining renewed public acceptance, although the exact nature and boundaries of transpersonal psychology are still being debated among academics.

Back in the realm of mainstream psychoanalysis, interest in thought-transference, unconscious communication, and even the paranormal continues to hover around current work on Ferenczi and Freud's papers on telepathy, as well as, more generally, in the work of such figures as the late Elizabeth Lloyd Mayer (2007) and the Jungian analyst Nathan Field (1991, 2006). While the place of these subjects within mainstream psychoanalytic thought remains ambiguous, I want to suggest that magical thinking has always been the motor driving psychoanalytic practice—an opinion with which many in the field would not, I suspect, be very eager to agree.

2

As June Bernstein (2002) reminds us, the word "magic" originally meant "of the magi"—the wise men of the Persians reputed to be skilled in enchantment. Definitions of magic include "any mysterious and overpowering quality that produces unaccountable or baffling effects," "the gratification of desires otherwise unobtainable," and "that which takes us beyond the ordinary action of cause and effect which we regard as natural" (p. 235). With this tripartite definition in mind, it seems clear that psychoanalysis is full of magical elements, especially in relation to the vicissitudes of the transference. The analytic encounter, with its deliberate quiet, low lighting, and use of the couch as a liminal space, specifically encourages the evocation of magic. Although Freud increasingly seemed to advocate the elimination of magic from psychoanalysis, plenty of magical elements remain in his theory and clinical practice. As Joel Whitebook argues (2002), the ambition completely to exorcise "enchantment" from human experience was one of the more misguided excesses of the Enlightenment.

In *Totem and Taboo* (1913), Freud explains that "the assumptions of magic are more fundamental and older than the doctrine of spirits, which forms the kernel of animism" (p. 91). Magic, according to Freud, is "the technique of animism" that "reveals in the clearest and most unmistakable way an intention to impose the laws governing mental life upon real things" (p. 91). Recent research suggests that otherwise rational people often act as though they believe they possess magical powers (though they may rationally deny it), a phenomenon that may be traceable to basic cognitive errors involving the perception of causal relationships. This kind of magical thinking occurs particularly in times of uncertainty or stress and serves our need for control, especially our need to perceive ourselves as able to navigate a clear path through overwhelming situations. Support for this explanation comes from studies showing that people display signs of magical thinking when they are faced with a combination of uncertainty about an outcome and a desire for control over that outcome (e.g., Bleak & Frederick, 1998; Friedland et al., 1992; Keinan, 1994; Matute, 1994). Magical thinking has been documented among Germans at the period of high unemployment and political instability in between the wars (Padgett & Jorgensen, 1982); police officers with jobs that put them in dangerous situations (Corrigan et al., 1980); HIV-infected men with no agency over their health (Taylor et al., 2000); and lottery players who possess "illusions of control" regarding their ability to influence chance wagers (Langer, 1975). Even when people recognize that control over life events may be impossible to achieve, magical beliefs may arise out of a motivation to find "meaning" in that which they cannot control (Pepitone & Saffiotti, 1997). It is well known, too, that magical thinking has equally magical results. Patients with metastasized cancer mysteriously go into remission and make miraculous recoveries. Experiments with placebos show that people have the power within them to produce all the effects of drugs, both benefits and side effects.

3

Freud always insisted that occult phenomena obeyed the same principles that underlie the psychodynamics of dreams, neurotic symptoms, and primary process thinking in general, characterized by the absence of "adult," ego-generated logic and order and a lack of attention to such factors as time, money, and duty. Clearly, these hallmarks of adult reality have no place in the magical world of the unconscious. As Freud acknowledged in his work on dreams, primary process thinking is timeless. In our dreams, split seconds last for an eternity, years pass in seconds, and chronologies are scrambled or reversed. This is the realm of myth, fairytales, and folklore, in which everyone is immortal. As Edmund Bergler and Géza Róheim (1946) put it,

> Time perception is an artifact built in the unconscious ego after the partial mastering of blows against the "autarchic fiction." Therefore time and duty are associated. In every endeavor in which childlike omnipotence is fantasied, normal perception of time is disturbed.
>
> (p. 197)

The inability to react or respond in an "adult," ego-directed way to time (and money) is also, of course, a classic hallmark of mental illness.

Not unsurprisingly, time and money are key subjects in the psychoanalytic encounter, where they take on a symbolic weight very different from that which they bear in "reality." This fact suggests that psychoanalysis takes place, at least in part, in the realm of magical thinking. Here, in this liminal world without shape or form, the ordinary proximity between two minds is narrowed and distorted, and mysterious transmissions can occur. Secrets make their way from one mind to another, sometimes without the use of words. On the couch, patients behave in magical ways, bringing the past alive in the present and merging with absent others. Psychoanalysts, too, act like magicians by offering themselves as contemporary objects to which the "ghosts" of the patient's past can attach themselves, thereby initiating the process of transference. The appearance of these ghosts in the analytic session allows both analysts and patients to become familiar with them, and even to become, as Auden (1939) put it, "enthusiastic over the night … for the sense of wonder it alone has to offer" (see also McDougall, 1985, p. 276). Regular exposure to the magic of the analytic session serves to disempower these ghosts of the past so that eventually, as Hans Loewald (1960) explains, they can be "laid to rest as ancestors" (p. 10). Their power is then available to be "taken over and transformed into the new intensity of present life, of the secondary process and contemporary objects" (pp. 248–249; see also McDougall, 1985, pp. 285–286).

Freud (1919) felt that people feared psychoanalysis because there was something uncanny about it. What they really feared, he speculated, was the area of their minds over which they have no control: the unconscious. Patients are reluctant to use the couch, explained Freud, because they fear giving up ordinary social reality and turning themselves over to the power of another way of being. The analyst creates the conditions (low lights, couch, quiet), for the emergence of magic (or at least, of magical thinking). From this perspective, psychoanalysis can be regarded, like magic, as a ritual to produce astonishment, a way to catalyze the phantasm.

4

In explaining how psychoanalysis "works," analysts often appeal to "experience," arguing that one can truly understand the effect of the process only by undergoing it, with the aid of an experienced analyst. This reliance on a specialist elite, initiated into occult knowledge, who proceed according to an essentially intuitive method, inspired much criticism in the early days of psychoanalysis.

Like most magic, that of psychoanalysis assumes the visible world is merely the outward manifestation of invisible forces and energies. It takes for granted the idea that life in the everyday world is actually contingent on the operations of a secret, "inner" reality not accessible to the senses; it also assumes that only very rare individuals can master this hidden knowledge. Such mastery is a source of great power, since to understand the workings of the secret forces implies the ability to change them.

To become an adept, in psychoanalysis as in magic, the neophyte must first learn to dissociate him- or herself from the "natural attitude" of laymen; only then can he or she begin a lengthy training, under close supervision by a designated sage who has special sight into the obscure dimension. Over many years and at great cost, the neophyte learns esoteric skills in dealing with invisible forces (transference, projection, and so on), becoming acquainted with a world not known to the senses (including "common sense"), far beyond the range of "ordinary" knowledge. Both magic and psychoanalysis encompass a bewildering variety of groups, branches, and systems of belief, each with its own history, masters, and particular rituals; and each branch is dominated by a small, rarified group of elders, mostly male, whose private lives, outside of the particular space and time of their practice, largely remain a secret. Both are mysterious realms of thought that can be understood only by the illuminated, whose practitioners in some way concern themselves with things that sociologist Marcello Truzzi (1971), in an essay on the dimensions and definitions of the occult, describes as anomalous to our generally accepted "cultural storehouse of truths" (p. 639).

One of the reasons why there is so much resistance to acknowledging the role played by magical thinking in the analytic encounter is that, according to anthropologists, this is the most primitive mode of thought, which, in the course of human phylogeny, has been followed by religious thinking, and finally, by scientific and analytical thinking (Frazer, 1890; Mauss, 1950). Indirect evidence for this claim comes from studies showing that people who have paranormal beliefs are somewhat less inclined to critical thinking than others (Brugger & Graves, 1997; Epstein et al., 1996; Pacini & Epstein, 1999); and this issue is explored in depth by Freud in *Totem and Taboo* (1913).

It would be wrong, however, to assume that development in cognition is a one-dimensional process, with magical thinking on the one end and analytical reasoning on the other. In fact, we all have many different modes of processing information, which, for the sake of convenience, may be divided into two kinds: the intuitive and the analytic. These rely on different areas in the brain, and have different rules of operation (Evans, 2003; Sloman, 1996; Stanovich & West, 2000; Sun et al., 2005). Jonathan Evans's (2003) research into dual-process thinking, for example, suggests the presence of "two minds in one brain" (p. 458): the rational, problem-solving stream of consciousness that Evans describes as "System 2 thinking," and, underlying this kind of thought, "a whole set of autonomous subsystems in System 1 that post only their final products into consciousness and compete directly for our inferences, decisions and actions" (p. 458). This set of subsystems might be referred to in layman's terms as intuitive thinking. Contrary to popular thought, critical thinking does not replace intuition as the mind matures; rather, as Evans suggests, both types of thinking continue to exist and develop throughout an individual's life. Therefore, people can hold conflicting beliefs that are rational and verbally justifiable on the one hand ("every number has an equal chance of winning the lottery"), and automatically resistant to logical arguments on the other ("my lucky number has a greater chance than any other").

The coexistence of two cognitive systems in the human brain is consistent with the classic claim that believers of magic and religion conceive of two different realities, a natural and a mystical reality (Bronowski, 1974; Lévy-Brühl, 1949; Tambiah, 1990). The mystical reality is thought to "unveil" when a person experiences something interpreted as mystical (Lévy-Brühl, 1949). Nevertheless, anxiety about occultism within the scientific community is not altogether without basis. Popular assumptions about those who believe in psychic powers have been borne out, some feel, by empirical studies showing that those especially inclined to paranormal beliefs generally use more intuitive (i.e., noncritical) thinking in everyday life (Epstein et al., 1996; Wolfradt et al., 1999). Furthermore, although differences between them are small, believers in the paranormal have been shown to be slightly less emotionally stable than skeptics (Wiseman & Watt, 2004). However, the same is true for those who believe in religion—a category that includes plenty of scientists among its ranks.

5

Ever since the death of Freud—but especially over the last 30 years—a significant amount of intellectual energy has been expended in attempts to give an account of the relation between psychoanalysis and science. These discussions have been protracted and involved, and it is not my project to recite them at any length here. What needs to be established, however, is that the way we think about psychoanalytic treatment today has changed significantly from Freud's model of the analyst as surgical, abstracted observer to what Robert Wallerstein (1998) describes as "a two-person psychology focused on the always subjective interactions of the transferential internalized object relationships of the patient with the countertransferential (or equally transferential) internalized object relations of the analyst" (pp. 1021–1022). Since 1923, the influence of Ferenczi and the entire tradition of object relations theory has provided an alternative model to Freud's "surgical" example of a self rooted in biology and motivated by unconscious physiological drives. In other words, the analyst's subjectivity is no longer regarded as something that should be kept as objective as possible, but cultivated as a primary tool of knowledge through empathic identification with the patient. When the discipline is reformulated in this light, we need to reconsider whether psychoanalysis can still be seen, as Freud saw it, as a "natural science," or whether it should be seen as more of a social-behavioral science, or as no longer a science at all, but a historical, cultural, or philosophical discipline, as many influential scholars and clinicians have argued, including Gill (1994), Wolff (1996), Crews (1995), and Phillips (1997).

A full account of the many approaches to this problem is given in the final chapter of Peter Rudnytsky's *Reading Psychoanalysis* (2002). Here, Rudnytsky argues that, while this new formulation of psychoanalysis as a mode of therapy makes it a hermeneutic discipline (and thus not bound by the canons of natural science), psychoanalysis as an interpretive practice "should be based on a theoretical foundation where such restrictive canons are both necessary and appropriate" (p. 202). Closing the divide between hermeneutic and scientific practices, he makes the case that psychoanalysis is not autonomous, isolated from the other sciences, both natural and human, but is sited at the crossroads between the two, marking the areas that both have in common, respecting both the claims of science as a theory, and the claims of the individual as a therapeutic practice.

A scholar who would clearly agree with this view of the analytic field was the physician, psychiatrist, and parapsychologist Jule Eisenbud (1908–99). Eisenbud was a graduate of the New York Psychoanalytic Institute and an associate clinical professor of psychiatry at the University of Colorado Medical School. He was a charter member of the Parapsychological Association and wrote numerous articles on psychiatry and psychoanalysis based on his experiments with telepathy, but he came to prominence largely through his book *The World of Ted Serios* (1967). In this book, he described his work with Serios, a Chicago bellhop, who had the uncanny ability to produce "thoughtographs," dream-like images of his thoughts, on film. Eisenbud's colleagues, however, found his work less exciting. A review of the Ted Serios book by Hans Eysenck (1967) in the *New York Times* concluded that "Dr. Eisenbud seems to have little notion of what experiments are and less liking for the rigors and methodological niceties of scientific research" (p. 20).

Although he was interested in psychic phenomena as a young man, and recalls reading Freud's "Dreams and Occultism," from the *New Introductory Lectures* (1933), during his medical internship, Eisenbud (1946) initially remained ambivalent about the existence of the paranormal. It was not until he had "painfully worked through" his resistance to the material he began to encounter in his own analytic practice that he "was able to appreciate the penetrating insights into telepathy that Freud presented in his *New Introductory Lectures*" (p. 10). He was also deeply impressed and strongly influenced by J. W. Dunne's *An Experiment with Time* (1927), an influential book about precognitive dreams.

Upon setting up in private practice, Eisenbud discovered that, almost from the beginning, his patients began to provide him with "striking examples of dreams and associations to which the telepathy hypothesis was reasonably applicable." He writes: "It was as if psychoanalysis, exciting and demanding enough as it was, had suddenly become multidimensional … [and] opened up a vast subterranean landscape that I had never dreamed existed" (1987, p. 11).

Eisenbud suggests that most analysts unconsciously develop a rigid reaction-formation against their more primitive tendencies:

> The so-called occult is no threat to us when we can view it with the comfortable assurance that it has no reality beyond that of the dramatic device. When it brushes by us in life itself, we have another problem on our hands entirely.
>
> (1946, p. 84)

Eisenbud convincingly argues that the psychoanalytic community is especially hardheaded and skeptical when it comes to the paranormal because most analysts rigidly isolate and dissociate individual events, repressing and defending whatever they cannot examine hypercritically. He proposes that the refusal of most psychoanalysts "to face certain facts full on, in all their implications" is "a defensive maneuver that allows business as usual to go on in the rest of one's life" (1967, p. 156), which is especially ironic given that, as Eisenbud suggests, these defenses may be an integral part of the mechanism that gives rise to paranormal events in the first place.

Eisenbud often reiterated (e.g., 1967, Chapter 15) his belief that everyone is capable of thought-transference, and we may, in fact, be using it unconsciously all the time. In other words, like Freud, he believed that thought-transference was not an isolated, dissociated form of perception, but part of the human personality, a current of life in tune with all the rest of our homeostatic needs. According to Eisenbud, this form of communication was just one of the many complex facets of the unconscious, and in his 1946 paper "Telepathy and the Problems of Psychoanalysis," published in the *Psychoanalytic Quarterly*, he endeavored to explain its method:

> The organism always acts with utmost economy of function, and the telepathic process can generally be observed to utilize whatever ordinary stepping stones lie to hand; but there comes a moment, just as when two electrodes approach that distance from each other at which the potential is

> able to snap the current across the intervening gap, when the spark occurs, and one can retrospectively observe that to achieve this spark, the patient, the analyst, or both—as influenced by some unseen force—have been pulled slightly (sometimes greatly) out of line with their expected individual orbits. (p. 86)

Other analysts sympathetic to this position include Mintz (1983), Fodor (1951), and Pederson-Krag (1947). Where Eisenbud's stance differs significantly from those of others working in the field, however, is in his firm conviction that paranormal events *have* long been proven to be scientifically valid: "the existence of telepathic functioning already rests on a foundation as firm as anything in the realm of empirical science" (1946, p. 83). Many, I imagine, would disagree with this statement, and likewise with his claim that "we do not today have to align ourselves with discredited crystal gazers and table-lifters; we are amply supported by researchers of the highest academic standing" (p. 86). "All in all," Eisenbud argues, "psychoanalysts may be assured that the study of so-called paranormal psychological phenomena can only strengthen that view of man and nature which science in general and psychoanalysis in particular has revealed to us" (p. 87). He finds it baffling that what he regards to be "the wide-ranging data" on thought-transference and other paranormal procedures (within the field of parapsychology) are totally excluded from the domain from which psychoanalysis draws its case studies, theories, and evidence, and he believes the psychoanalytic prejudice against "paranormal" phenomena would be considerably undermined if analysts looked at the nonanalytic literature on the subject, especially at the data provided in standard works in the field of parapsychology.

Eisenbud is referring here to the Rhine experiments, summarized in the book *Extra-Sensory Perception after Sixty Years* (Rhine et al., 1940. In the late 1930s, psychologist J. B. Rhine, along with his colleague William McDougall, conducted an extensive series of experiments in parapsychology at Duke University. By 1940, Rhine and his team had accumulated a series of 33 experiments, involving almost a million trials, with protocols that rigorously excluded possible sensory clues. Twenty-seven of the 33 studies produced statistically significant results. Furthermore, positive results were not restricted only to Rhine's lab. In the five years following Rhine's first publication of his results, 33 independent replication experiments were conducted at different laboratories; 61% of these were statistically significant, where a total of 5% would have been expected by chance alone.

Even today, scholars such as Susan Lazar (2001) complain that a skeptical attitude persists toward psychic phenomena "despite robust evidence demonstrating the reality of nonlocal phenomena such as telepathy and the impact of mind from a distance" (p. 114). Yet it is crucial to remember that, according to mainstream scientific thought, no such "robust evidence" exists. The Rhine experiments, although evaluated by the most rigorous statistical methods, used enormous numbers of subjects and huge numbers of guesses, and, as a result, have always been considered suspicious and controversial by the scientific establishment. More recently, the U.S. National Academy of Sciences published a 1988 report on the subject, concluding there is "no scientific justification from research conducted over a period of 130 years for the existence of parapsychological phenomena" (Druckman & Swets, 1988, p. 22). In 1991, in a survey of opinion among scientists in the National Academy of Sciences, 96% described themselves as "skeptical" of ESP (McConnell & Clark, 1991). Finally, a recent study using neuroimaging is believed to "provide the strongest evidence yet obtained that paranormal mental phenomena do not exist" (Moulton & Kosslyn, 2008, p. 182). It seems fair to say, then, that the scientific community has rejected all claims of psychic phenomena, since, according to the accepted criteria, no compelling evidence of such phenomena has yet been found.

6

Psychoanalytic practice is devoted to the exploration of the individual, in a certain place and for a certain amount of time, which means that truly repeatable experiments are inherently impossible, since no two individuals are alike. It defies the ethos of psychoanalytic practice to provide an objective measurement of its "results" (or even a subjective measurement, for that matter). The unconscious cannot even truly be described, since language is alien to the primary process, just as it often is to dreams, and the imagination in general. Indeed, any endeavor that is deeply reliant on symbolic thinking cannot, by definition, be strictly scientific—or even, for that matter, strictly rational.

"One of the most remarkable facts in the history of the psychoanalytic movement," wrote Jule Eisenbud in 1946, "is the indifference with which Freud's publications on the subject of telepathy were received." Eisenbud considered this neglect to be particularly significant in the light of "the obsessive, exegetical tendencies" (p. 85) of the early Freudians. In an essay written almost 40 years later, he was still acutely conscious of "the curious irony" that "the two disciplines which have most to do with unconscious factors in human affairs, parapsychology and psychoanalysis, have so little regard for each other, and play so little part in each other's thinking" (1967, p. 11). It can be safely said that, even today, most practitioners dislike analogies between psychoanalysis and the occult, which they are likely to find emotionally threatening or disturbing. In the preface to his monograph *Telepathy and Medical Psychology* (1947), Jan Ehrenwald remarks that, when he embarked on research into the paranormal, he was admonished "that whoever wants to expound his views on matters of psychical research would be best advised first to state his credentials" (p. 5). Things appear to have changed very little today, if they have changed at all.

Note

1 This chapter originally appeared as: Brottman, M. (2009). Psychoanalysis and magic: Then and now. *American Imago, 66*, 471–489. Reprinted with permission.

References

Auden, W. H. (1939). In memory of Sigmund Freud. In E. Mendelson (Ed.), *Collected poems* (pp. 273–276). Vintage Books.

Bergler, E., & Róheim, G. (1946). The psychology of time perception. *Psychoanalytic Quarterly*, 15, 190–206.

Bernstein, J. (2002). Magic in psychoanalysis. *Modern Psychoanalysis*, 27, 235–242.

Bleak, J. L., & Frederick, C. M. (1998). Superstitious behavior in sport: Levels of effectiveness and determinants of use in three collegiate sports. *Journal of Sport Behavior*, 21, 1–15.

Breuer, J., & Freud, S. (1895). Studies on hysteria. In J. Strachey (Ed. & Trans.), *The standard edition of the complete psychological works of Sigmund Freud* (Vol. 2, pp. 1–305). Hogarth Press.

Bronowski, J. (1974). *Magic, science, and civilization*. Columbia University Press.

Brugger, P., & Graves, R. E. (1997). Testing vs. believing hypotheses: Magical ideation in the judgment of contingencies. *Cognitive Neuropsychiatry*, 2, 251–272.

Chertok, L., & de Saussure, R. (1973). *The therapeutic revolution: From Mesmer to Freud* (R. H. Ahrenfeldt, Trans.). Brunner Mazel.

Corrigan, R. S., Pattison, L., & Lester, D. (1980). Superstition in police officers. *Psychological Reports*, 46, 830.

Crews, F. (1995). *The memory wars: Freud's legacy in dispute*. New York Review of Books.

Druckman, D., & Swets, J. A. (Eds.). (1988). *Enhancing human performance: Issues, theories and techniques*. National Academy Press.

Dunne, J. W. (1927). *An experiment with time*. A. & C. Black.

Ehrenwald, J. (1947). *Telepathy and medical psychology*. Norton.

Eisenbud, J. (1946). Telepathy and problems of psychoanalysis. *Psychoanalytic Quarterly*, 15, 82–87.

Eisenbud, J. (1967). *The world of Ted Serios: "Thoughtographic" studies of an extraordinary mind*. William Morrow.

Epstein, S., Pacini, R., Denes-Raj, V., & Heier, H. (1996). Individual differences in intuitive-experiential and analytical-rational thinking styles. *Journal of Personality and Social Psychology*, 71, 390–405.

Evans, J. S. B. T. (2003). In two minds: Dual-process accounts of reasoning. *Trends in Cognitive Science*, 7, 454–459.

Eysenck, H. (1967). Review of "The world of Ted Serios: 'Thoughtographic' studies of an extraordinary mind," by Jule Eisenbud. *The New York Times Book Review*, May 14, p. 20.

Field, N. (1991). Projective identification: Mechanism or mystery? *Journal of Analytical Psychology*, 36, 93–109.

Field, N. (2006). *Breakdown and breakthrough: Psychotherapy in a new dimension*. Routledge.

Fodor, N. (1951). *New approaches to dream interpretation*. Citadel Press.

Frazer, J. (1890). *The golden bough: A study in magic and religion* (R. Fraser, Ed.). Macmillan.

Freud, S. (1890). Psychical (or mental) treatment. In J. Strachey (Ed. & Trans.), *The standard edition of the complete psychological works of Sigmund Freud* (Vol. 7, pp. 283–302). Hogarth Press.

Freud, S. (1901). The psychopathology of everyday life. In J. Strachey (Ed. & Trans.), *The standard edition of the complete psychological works of Sigmund Freud* (Vol. 6, pp. 1–272). Hogarth Press.

Freud, S. (1912). A note on the unconscious in psychoanalysis. In J. Strachey (Ed. & Trans.), *The standard edition of the complete psychological works of Sigmund Freud* (Vol. 12, pp. 260–266). Hogarth Press.

Freud, S. (1913). Totem and taboo. In J. Strachey (Ed. & Trans.), *The standard edition of the complete psychological works of Sigmund Freud* (Vol. 13, pp. 1–161). Hogarth Press.

Freud, S. (1919). The "uncanny". In J. Strachey (Ed. & Trans.), *The standard edition of the complete psychological works of Sigmund Freud* (Vol. 17, pp. 219–252). Hogarth Press.

Freud, S. (1922). Some additional notes on dream interpretation as a whole: The occult significance of dreams. In J. Strachey (Ed. & Trans.), *The standard edition of the complete psychological works of Sigmund Freud* (Vol. 19, pp. 135–138). Hogarth Press.

Freud, S. (1933). New introductory lectures on psychoanalysis. In J. Strachey (Ed. & Trans.), *The standard edition of the complete psychological works of Sigmund Freud* (Vol. 22, pp. 7–182). Hogarth Press.

Friedland, N., Keinan, G., & Regev, Y. (1992). Controlling the uncontrollable: Effects of stress on illusory perceptions of controllability. *Journal of Personality and Social Psychology*, 63, 923–931.

Gill, M. (1994). *Psychoanalysis in transition: A personal view*. The Analytic Press.

Jones, E. (1957). *The life and work of Sigmund Freud* (Vol. 3). Basic Books.

Jung, C. G. (1961). *Memories, dreams, reflections* (A. Jaffé, Ed.; R. Winston & C. Winston, Trans.). Random House.

Keinan, G. (1994). Effects of stress and tolerance of ambiguity on magical thinking. *Journal of Personality and Social Psychology*, 67, 48–55.

Koutstaal, W. (1992). Skirting the abyss: A history of experimental explorations in automatic writing in psychology. *Journal of the History of the Behavioral Sciences*, 28, 5–27.

Kris, E. (1952). *Psychoanalytic explorations in art*. International Universities Press.

Langer, E. J. (1975). The illusion of control. *Journal of Personality and Social Psychology*, 32, 311–328.

Lazar, S. G. (2001). Knowing, influencing, and healing: Paranormal phenomena and implications for psychoanalysis and psychotherapy. *Psychoanalytic Inquiry*, 21, 113–132.

Lévy-Brühl, L. (1949). *The notebooks on primitive mentality* (P. Rivière, Trans.). Blackwell.

Loewald, H. (1960). On the therapeutic action of psychoanalysis. In *Papers on psychoanalysis* (pp. 221–256). Yale University Press.

Mauss, M. (1950). *A general theory of magic* (R. Brain, Trans.). Routledge.

Matute, H. (1994). Learned helplessness and superstitious behavior as opposite effects of uncontrollable reinforcement in humans. *Learning and Motivation*, 25, 216–232.

Mayer, E. L. (2007). *Extraordinary knowing: Science, skepticism, and the inexplicable powers of the human mind*. Bantam.

McConnell, R. A., & Clark, T. K. (1991). National Academy of Sciences' opinion on parapsychology. *Journal of the American Society for Psychical Research*, 85, 333–365.
McDougall, J. (1985). *Theaters of the mind: Illusion and truth on the psychoanalytic stage*. Basic Books.
Mintz, E. E. (1983). *The psychic thread: Paranormal and transpersonal aspects of psychotherapy*. Human Sciences Press.
Moulton, S. T., & Kosslyn, S. M. (2008). Using neuroimaging to resolve the psi debate. *Journal of Cognitive Neuroscience*, 20, 182–192.
Noll, R. (1997). *The Jung cult: Origins of a charismatic movement*. Free Press.
Pacini, R., & Epstein, S. (1999). The relation of rational and experiential information-processing styles to personality, basic beliefs, and the ratio-bias phenomenon. *Journal of Personality and Social Psychology*, 76, 972–987.
Padgett, V. R., & Jorgensen, D. O. (1982). Superstition and economic threat: Germany 1918–1940. *Personality and Social Psychology Bulletin*, 8, 736–741.
Pederson-Krag, G. (1947). Telepathy and repression. *Psychoanalytic Quarterly*, 16, 61–68.
Pepitone, A., & Saffiotti, L. (1997). The selectivity of nonmaterial beliefs in interpreting life events. *European Journal of Social Psychology*, 27, 23–35.
Phillips, A. (1997). *Terrors and experts*. Harvard University Press.
Rhine, J. B., Pratt, J. G., Smith, B. M., Stuart, C. E., & Greenwood, J. A. (1940). *Extra-sensory perception after sixty years*. Humphries.
Rudnytsky, P. L. (2002). *Reading psychoanalysis: Freud, Rank, Ferenczi, Groddeck*. Cornell University Press.
Schwentker, W. (1987). Passion as a mode of life: Max Weber, the Otto Gross circle and eroticism. In W. J. Mommsen & J. Osterhammel (Eds.), *Max Weber and his contemporaries* (pp. 483–498). Harper Collins.
Shamdasani, S. (1993). Automatic writing and the discovery of the unconscious. *Spring*, 54, 100–131.
Sloman, S. A. (1996). The empirical case for two systems of reasoning. *Psychological Bulletin*, 119, 3–22.
Stanovich, K. E., & West, R. F. (2000). Individual differences in reasoning: Implications for the rationality debate? *Behavioral and Brain Sciences*, 23, 645–726.
Sun, R., Slusarz, P., & Terry, C. (2005). The interaction of the explicit and the implicit in skill learning: A dual-process approach. *Psychological Review*, 112, 159–192.
Swales, P. J. (1986). Freud, his teacher, and the birth of psychoanalysis. In P. E. Stepansky (Ed.), *Freud: Appraisals and reappraisals* (Vol. 1, pp. 2–82). The Analytic Press.
Tambiah, S. J. (1990). *Magic, science, religion, and the scope of rationality*. Cambridge University Press.
Taylor, S. E., Kemeny, M. E., Reed, G. M., Bower, J. E., & Gruenewald, T. L. (2000). Psychological resources, positive illusions, and health. *American Psychologist*, 55, 99–109.
Truzzi, M. (1971). Definition and dimensions of the occult: Towards a sociological perspective. *Journal of Popular Culture*, 5, 637–648.
Wallerstein, R. M. (1998). The new American psychoanalysis: A commentary. *Journal of the American Psychoanalytic Association*, 46, 1021–1043.
Whitebook, J. (2002). Slow magic: Psychoanalysis and "The disenchantment of the world". *Journal of the American Psychoanalytic Association*, 50, 1197–1218.
Wiseman, R., & Watt, C. (2004). Measuring superstitious belief: Why lucky charms matter. *Personality and Individual Differences*, 37, 1533–1541.

Wolff, P. H. (1996). The irrelevance of infant observations for psychoanalysis. *Journal of the American Psychoanalytic Association*, 44, 369–392.

Wolfradt, U., Oubaid, V., Straube, E. R., Bischoff, N., & Mischo, J. (1999). Thinking styles, schizotypal traits, and anomalous experiences. *Personality and Individual Differences*, 27, 821–830.

Chapter 13

Rethinking Telepathy

Thomas Rabeyron

We end this collection with an exposition by the French psychoanalyst and parapsychologist Thomas Rabeyron, whose joint publication in the Journal of the American Psychoanalytic Association *provided the impetus to creating this group of psychoanalysts and this book. Not only does Thomas discuss a number of telepathic communications in psychoanalysis, but then—turning to Bion and Balint—he posits that there is a primordial "ontic" order—the Bionian "O"—from which telepathic phenomena derive. He concludes that within this order "the ordinary laws of space, time, and causality do not operate in the way we usually experience them" and that this accounts for the trepidation which psychoanalysts (and people in general) have about accepting these phenomena. This final chapter also represents a plea to those in the fields of psychoanalysis and parapsychology to continue to explore together.*

* * * *

Spontaneous Telepathic Experiences and Laboratory Experiments about Psi

Telepathic experiences belong to the domain of exceptional occurrences (Rabeyron, 2020a), with some people spontaneously reporting situations in which they have the impression of direct access to another person's thoughts. Sally Rhine-Feather and Michael Schmicker (2005) compiled numerous accounts of such telepathic perceptions, and they presented cases where people reported "sensing" from a distance when a loved one was in danger—as in the following case:

> One Sunday afternoon, several members of our family were eating at my paternal grandmother's house. Suddenly, and for no apparent reason in the midst of pleasant family dinner chatter, my mother stood up and screamed, "My mother! My mother! Something has happened to my mother!" We were all shocked … About fifteen minutes after her experience, the phone rang, and she received the information from her father that her mother had

DOI: 10.4324/9781003611042-14

> indeed died fifteen minutes previously. My mother was not aware that her mother was ill, or even that she was in a hospital, where she expired.
>
> (p. 26)

The authors conclude:

> The ordinary hallucination produces fantasy, nonsense and verifiably false claims and usually occurs in people who are mentally or physically ill or in a drugged state. The Extra Sensory Perception (ESP) hallucination delivers accurate, factual information that is subsequently checked out, verified and is experienced by sane, healthy, normal people.
>
> (p. 28)

Here are two similar cases coming from my clinical practice (Rabeyron, 2020a; Rabeyron et al., 2020):

> After not seeing her mother for several weeks, Marion suddenly felt a sharp pain in her chest and told her husband, "It squeezes me. It hurts too much." She then thought of her mother, who as far as she knew was not ill. Marion later receives a call from her brother telling her that their mother had died of a heart attack at that time.
>
> Paula relates a dream in which her boyfriend, a soldier, is wearing his army uniform, with a black beret, the meaning of which she does not know. He tells her that he loves her, that he is leaving, but that he will always be close to her and that she should not be sad. Then, Paula wakes up and sees that it is 7:15 in the morning. She will learn later that her boyfriend, while abroad, has died around the same time that day.

These experiences may be reported by patients about events that have occurred outside the analytical session, but they also emerge in the psychoanalytical setting. We may first consider them to be the result of an incidental encounter between the patient's unconscious death wish and events occurring simultaneously, which might occur for purely statistical reasons. Yet accounts of such events, and their emergence in analysis, are sometimes so precise that such a hypothesis appears difficult to sustain. Some cases of ostensibly telepathic experiences only seem to become intelligible when we consider the possibility of some kind of "interactions at a distance." Many questions then arise: Why do some people report such experiences? What is the ontological status of these phenomena? And what might psychoanalysis say about these "objective" aspects of telepathy?

Regarding the first question, a substantial body of psychological research explores the conditions under which exceptional and telepathic experiences arise (Cardeña et al., 2000). Most individuals report such unusual experiences following difficult life circumstances, traumatic events, or other significant stressors (Rabeyron & Watt, 2010). Exceptional experiences like telepathy can thus be understood as part of a "paranormal solution" (Rabeyron, 2020a), emerging as a psychological response to encounters at the boundaries of subjective experience. When we seek to understand why certain individuals develop such a solution, we see that these individuals often report specific configurations of early intersubjective relationships (intrusive, controlling, unpredictable, distant, etc.) and various traumatic experiences later in childhood. In this context, exceptional experiences appear to serve several functions (Rabeyron, 2020a; Rabeyron & Loose, 2015). First, they offer a representational system that provides an illusion of control over the environment, rooted in omnipotence and magical thinking ("the pathway of control"). Then they also allow for the expression of imaginary elements and various forms of beliefs linked to the paranormal ("the pathway of imagination"). Moreover, they often emerge within family environments steeped in paranormal themes and, more broadly, lead to the expression of transgenerational contents whose strange and unsettling nature is frequently associated with psychic concerns around grief and death ("the pathway of transmission").

These different processual pathways are embedded within a personality structure that facilitates the emergence of such experiences. The main characteristic of this structure is an exacerbated "psychic permeability" (Hartmann, 1991) and "transliminality" (Thalbourne, 2000), which foster experiences perceived as unusual in their environment. These individuals often describe themselves as "sponges" or "bubbles," reflecting a fragile "skin-ego" and a high level of porosity to primary processes (Anzieu, 1974, 1993). They thus report a certain sensitivity that combines intuition and hyper-empathy, alongside a psychic functioning marked by projective identification. This manifests according to a "two-faced" logic, oscillating between conscious and unconscious processes, internal and external worlds, but also in a "bidirectional" manner, resulting in both perceptive and projective movements. More generally, exceptional experiences can be understood as the expression of an extreme form of the symbolization process showcasing its most primordial levels (Rabeyron & Loose, 2015). A detailed study of certain exceptional experiences thus provides deeper insights into the fundamental coordinates of subjective experience (Rabeyron, 2023). In this regard, telepathy questions certain forms of primordial communication within the domain of "chimeras" (De M'Uzan, 1977) and "co-thinking" (Widlöcher, 1996). The undifferentiated forms of communication that emerge in this context, closest to the real, the body, and the other, offer an original perspective on the nature of a primordial intersubjectivity (Rabeyron et al., 2020; Tennes, 2007).

Regarding the ontological status of telepathy, there is a longstanding tradition of intellectual inquiry within the field of psychical research (Méheust, 1999). As Bertrand Méheust (1999) and Régine Plas (2000) have noted, many of Freud's[1] contemporaries—prominent figures within the intellectual establishment—considered that telepathy contains a "kernel of truth" among occult claims. These included influential thinkers such as Bergson, James, Gödel, Richet, Durkheim, and Jaurès. If thought-transference was to correspond to a genuine interaction beyond usual spatial and temporal boundaries, it would not only expand the scope of possible analytical interpretations, but also carry significant implications for psychoanalytic epistemology. In this regard, telepathic processes might be catalyzed by the analytical situation due to the strength of the affective bond between the analyst and the analysand and the regression processes induced by the setting, two significant factors in the emergence of supposed telepathic phenomena. For example, Balint (1955) noted:

> I too have had in my practice a few cases of apparent telepathy which, even after careful examination, have remained inexplicable by the mechanisms mentioned above. For quite a while I collected these cases without doing anything about them, in the hope that sooner or later I should understand them better. Quite gradually, it then dawned upon me that in all cases of this kind there was a particular emotional situation between the analyst and his patient.
>
> (p. 32)

Servadio (1935), Eisenbud (1966), and Ehrenwald (1971, 1978) have also analyzed material gathered through both clinical analysis and experimental studies. Ullman et al. (1973) conducted sleep laboratory experiments to investigate potential instances of dream telepathy. In exploring the possible reality of telepathy, these analysts were compelled to re-examine their conceptual frameworks, seeking to better understand psi phenomena and their integration within the dynamics of transference. One of the best-known contemporary analysts who has worked on this topic is Robert Stoller (Mayer, 2001), whose objective was to "stimulate a process of what he calls responsible data collecting concerning apparently anomalous, possibly telepathic experiences" (p. 631), experiences including "seemingly telepathic dreams" that appeared "more than coincidental" (p. 635). Stoller explained:

> I am not intrigued with the subject of telepathy nor a devotee of that literature, usually feeling the reports I chance upon to be foolish or fraud. Having finally decided to present these data, I shall not like having directed at me the sort of derogatory thoughts I often have when others broach the subject. But the data—seemingly telepathic dreams—appear more than coincidental; perhaps it is time to take a look.
>
> (p. 635)

Stoller went on to report some interesting examples of telepathy with his patients, taking in particular the form of telepathic dreams. Contemporary psychoanalytic literature contains similar situations of telepathic phenomenon (see, for example, Brottman, 2011; de Peyer, 2014, 2016, 2017; Eshel, 2006, 2010, 2012, 2019; Helm, 2018; Papazian, 2017; Reichbart, 2019; Rosenbaum, 2011; Tennes, 2007), which question the usual limits of the ego. They also challenge the boundaries of consciousness experiences and their relationship to space and time.

These observations from analytical studies are supported by a number of experiments examining telepathic phenomena under controlled conditions (Cardeña, 2018; Cardeña et al., 2015; Radin, 2010, 2018). The Ganzfeld protocol is the most widely used experimental setting for studying telepathy (Bem & Honorton, 1994). In this experience, the participant—referred to as the "percipient"—is seated comfortably while listening to white noise and viewing a uniform visual field through a mask. This sensory environment induces a modified state of consciousness, facilitating the emergence of hypnagogic hallucinations. The percipient then attempts to identify, from a set of target images, the one that has been "transmitted" telepathically by a second participant, known as the "agent" or "transmitter," who is located in a separate room. Studies utilizing the Ganzfeld protocol have produced dozens of scientific publications and several meta-analyses (Storm et al., 2010), yielding statistically significant results that suggest the ontological existence of thought-transference.

As psychology professor Deborah Delanoy (2005) notes: "By scientific standards, these meta-analyses establish that 'something' is happening in these studies. But is this 'something' psi or, as some critics have argued, more simply, unrecognized statistical problems or undetected methodological artifacts?" (p. 59). The current state of research on telepathy thus remains marked by divergent interpretations and an ongoing lack of scientific consensus (Alcock et al., 2003). Some scholars adopt a skeptical perspective, attributing positive results to fraud or undetected methodological errors (Wiseman, 2010). Others acknowledge that the findings suggest a genuine form of perception (Radin, 2010, 2018). A third perspective, which we will develop later in this chapter, sees these results as indicative of interactions beyond conventional models of information transfer, proposing instead that they reflect some kind of "entanglement" (Rabeyron, 2020b; Lucadou et al., 2007).

Ultimately, it appears undeniable that "something" has been observed under controlled conditions using reliable experimental methodologies. This has led some researchers in the field to advocate for a more open-minded approach to telepathy and its potential implications for our understanding of consciousness. Likewise, several psychoanalysts have argued that clinicians should consider the implication of these findings in their practice. Elizabeth Mayer (2001) pointed out that "significant experimental research has accumulated in recent years to suggest that telepathy … may constitute a real and scientifically verifiable phenomenon" (p. 634), while Lazar (2001) explains that "it would appear likely that sooner or later the fields of psychotherapy and psychoanalysis will be obliged to confront and to struggle to integrate robust research findings with respect to paranormal ways of knowing" (p. 129).

Functions of Telepathic Phenomena in the Analytical Setting

The psychoanalytic setting appears to facilitate telepathic experiences, likely due to states of regression and the dynamics of transference. This underscores the importance of recognizing and understanding such experiences within clinical practice and questions the potential "functions" of telepathy in the psychoanalytical setting. In this regard, following Freud's (1921, 1922, 1925, 1933) early hypotheses, several authors have interpreted thought-transference as the resurgence of primary intersubjective relations and a return to an archaic mode of communication (Papazian, 2017; Tennes, 2007). Numerous telepathic phenomena have also been observed within the mother–infant dyad, suggesting that the analytic relationship may, in some ways, evoke a similar relational dynamic between analyst and analysand. Ehrenwald (1978) and Balint (1955) similarly viewed thought-transference as an attempt by the patient to re-establish a connection with the analyst akin to the early mother–child relationship. Expanding on this idea, Mayer (2007) and Stoller (Mayer, 2001) proposed that such phenomena might stem from the analysand's unconscious longing for a primordial, preverbal connection with the analyst.

Conversely, other analysts have observed that the emergence of thought-transference in psychoanalysis may be linked to a "failure" in the intimate connection between analyst and analysand. Servadio (1958) proposed this hypothesis to explain patients' telepathic experiences and dreams, suggesting that such phenomena arise when the usual channels of communication are disrupted. Then, for Stoller (Mayer, 2001), what matters is not the content of telepathic thought but rather its container—that is, the analysand's desperate attempt to maintain a psychic bond with the analyst, particularly during or after a period of separation (Papazian, 2017). This, he argued, is a key factor in the emergence of telepathic dreams. Similarly, Reiner (2004) and Chaperot (2011) suggest that patients might use thought-transference as a way to recapture the analyst's attention if they perceive the latter as mentally absent during a session. In such cases, telepathic occurrences often manifest as striking coincidences between the analysand's words and the analyst's unspoken thoughts, suddenly re-engaging the analyst in the session. This idea aligns with Hann-Kende's (1953) insight that telepathic manifestations can emerge when the analyst's investment of the analysand diminishes. Along these lines, Prados (1959) argued that telepathic processes are more likely to occur when the patient senses a threat of separation, particularly when they feel that the analyst lacks empathy. Thus, telepathy in the analytic setting could be understood as an unconscious mechanism for preserving or restoring a vital psychic connection when it is perceived as weakened or at risk.

Telepathic processes in analysis may be linked more specifically to the early mother–child relationship in cases of traumatic experiences and an absent mother. In such instances, the patient seeks to establish a primary connection with the analyst through a form of telepathic transference, reviving an early mode of communication within the analytic setting. Balint (1955) describes these occurrences—what he terms "telepathic feats" (p. 119)—as especially prevalent in patients with affective deficiencies. For these patients, thought-transference represents an idealized form of connection, an unconscious attempt to repair early relational ruptures

(Kohut, 1972). Balint further suggests that telepathic phenomena are most likely to emerge when the patient experiences an intense positive transference, an observation echoed by Ansell (1966) and Löfgren (1968), who propose that telepathy might compensate for failures in early relationships. In the same perspective, Mayer (2007) notes that patients presenting apparent telepathy "believed that they had developed their gifts in response to trauma, in order to survive circumstances that required knowing more than people can possibly know. Again, those patients said they *had* to know. They couldn't afford not to" (p. 101).

Similarly, Ofra Eshel (2006) interprets telepathic dreams as "a search engine to seek and find the analyst, in order to halt the process of abandonment and prevent a return and collapse into the depths of despair of the early traumatization" (p. 1620). Eshel hypothesizes that episodes of thought-transference occur particularly in patients who have been confronted with a "mother who is absent-within-presence" (p. 1620). Telepathic experiences are thus frequently reported by patients with narcissistic disorders who have developed a "dead mother complex" (Green, 1983). These experiences would allow the patient to communicate early traumas in the form of "chimeric darkness" (Eshel, 2012) shared with the analyst, an idea also emphasized by Reiner (2004), Bass (2004), Papazian (2017), and Sánchez-Medina (2018).

Telepathic events then evoke a "common fantasy of symbiotic communication" (Lévy, 2007) shaping the transferential dynamic. From the analysand's perspective, this remnant of the archaic relationship could be interpreted as a resistance to the separation from the mother, and the patient would re-enact his or her primary investments through transferential repetition. Chervet (2009) thus proposes to consider telepathy as an "anti-traumatic" solution opposing the de-objectification and the ensuing separation–individuation processes. According to Searles (1979), these "zones of functional symbiosis" would then have a therapeutic aim, favoring the reconstruction of psychic envelopes. Lévy (2007) proposes a similar hypothesis, suggesting that "this zone of symbiosis between analysand and analyst, by creating the all-powerful illusion of a possible identity between the object encountered and the object preformed by desire, precedes and aims to make accessible this work of mourning that opens up the subjectivating process of separation–individuation" (p. 191).

Two complementary processes may thus underlie the emergence of telepathic phenomena in analysis. First, the analytic setting fosters regression in both the analyst and the analysand, facilitating a mode of fusional functioning that aligns with a regressive-restorative process (Rizzolo, 2016). Patients who have experienced disruptions in early fusion-connection states may seek to reestablish such a bond with the analyst. However, for these same patients, an abrupt rupture of this fusional state could provoke telepathic phenomena as a desperate attempt to preserve or restore the lost sense of regression and union. This process, in turn, may also give rise to telepathic experiences linked to what Rizzolo (2016) describes as a "regressive-defensive" process, where telepathy serves as a psychic mechanism to counteract the perceived threat of separation.

Thought-transference can also be understood as the patient's attempt to assert control over the analytic relationship. In this dynamic, the apparent concordance of thoughts reverses the typical transferential relationship: The patient, attuned to the vulnerabilities inherent to the analytic situation, unconsciously "scrutinizes" the analyst's psyche, exposing repressed material of the analyst. Eisenbud (1970) argued that analyses of allegedly telepathic dreams often "spotlight with great specificity and precision something that the analyst is laboring to repress" (p. 364). In one case, he observed that "the patient might have been mirroring my own repressed destructive wishes toward my wife and her pregnancy" (p. 369). Similarly, Branfman and Bunker (1952) described instances in which patients appeared to access personal information about their analysts' lives and concerns. In this regard, Servadio (1958) and Prados (1959) suggested that analysts should closely examine their countertransference responses when telepathic experiences arise, as these may provide crucial insight into unconscious dynamics at play in which the patient reflects back to the analyst unelaborated psychic elements. Freud's (1933) reaction to a telepathic experience with the Wolf Man exemplifies this dynamic (Birot, 2016) in which telepathic experiences can induce astonishment, anxiety, and uncanny sensations into the analyst's mind. Similarly, Balint (1955) admitted reluctance to publish his own inexplicable cases, noting that they had occurred in moments of intense emotional tension. Thought-transference, in this sense, exposes the imperfections and uncertainties of the analyst, often carrying with it feelings of ambiguity and even shame. Its emergence in analysis may thus illuminate the more obscure aspects of countertransference, which could partly explain the persistent reluctance within the field to openly discuss this kind of phenomenon.

Telepathy and Analytical Practice

Taking the telepathic hypothesis seriously may then lead analysts to reconsider their stance on telepathic phenomena reported by analysands. This perspective has already been explored by many authors, especially Freud, Ferenczi, Hollós, Fodor, Balint, Servadio, Eisenbud, Ehrenwald, Ullman, and more recently by Brottman, de Peyer, Eshel, Helm, Reichbart, Papazian, Reiner, Rosenbaum, and Tennes. This calls for a global reflection on how clinical practice and theoretical models of psychoanalysis might evolve in order to integrate the telepathic hypothesis. Three levels of potential transformation within the analytic framework and practice can then be identified (Rabeyron et al., 2021), focusing on listening, interpretation, and what Bion (1965) refers to as O, considered as being the ineffable and ultimate reality underlying psychic experience.

- *Regarding listening*: The psychoanalytic approach is rooted in an ethos of unconditional acceptance and openness, guiding the subject toward a form of truth. As Freud repeatedly emphasized, psychoanalysis is a search for truth, and as such, the analyst must be attuned to the full spectrum of human experience, including aspects that seem incongruous or disturbing in relation to their understanding of their own psychic and external realities. A parallel could be drawn with gender identity, which can provoke intense transferential reactions, challenging the analyst's own perceptions of the gendered self. To dismiss such telepathic experiences as madness or illusion would block the analyst from truly embracing the patient's narrative. Yet as Mayer (2001) suggests, these experiences can profoundly impact the analyst's own psychic life. Should psychoanalysis not evolve in its approach to such phenomena, as it has in its evolving understanding of gender? As a science of subjectivity, should psychoanalysis not engage with all forms of truth, even those most challenging to the materialist and reductionist paradigms that dominate Western thought?

- *Regarding interpretation*: Once the analyst begins to consider the telepathic hypothesis seriously, his or her interpretation of patients' accounts may evolve. Telepathic dreams could be classically interpreted as the expressions of unconscious aggression, disguised as a seemingly paranormal experience. In this case, the analysis might center the interpretation on exploring these aggressive feelings. However, if we accept the telepathic hypothesis, the analyst might interpret the dream as a reflection of the patient's attachment and a deep concern or anxiety about someone else. The analysis would then focus on guiding the patient to elaborate and understand these concerns and the underlying anxieties. This shift in perspective raises further questions for the analyst: How should they interpret the "co-incidence" between the patient's narrative and their own psychic state? Should the analyst inform the patient that a dream relates to something the analyst has experienced? Would this revelation provoke astonishment or a deeper understanding in the analysand?
- *Regarding O*: The concept of O, introduced by Bion (1965), refers to the underlying nature of reality that remains beyond our direct access. It is akin to Kant's notion of the "thing-in-itself" (*Das Ding*) or Lacan's idea of The Real (*Le réel*). For Bion, O represents an ultimate, infinite, and unknowable truth that serves as the source of all transformational processes. In this context, the telepathic hypothesis reorients our understanding of the relationship between the analyst and the analysand, challenging the idea of a rigid boundary between them. The analytic situation creates a profound, intimate bond between both parties that transcends the interactions within the session itself, but what are the limits of this connection? Telepathic experiences could point to a deeper, transpersonal bond extending across both space and time, suggesting a shared psychic reality that blurs the lines between subject and object. This prospect may evoke significant concern in the analyst, as it implies that the psychoanalytic framework, which traditionally protects the analyst from the full psychic reality of the analysand, may only offer partial defense. As Balint (1955) notes, such concerns could explain the reluctance to explore telepathy: Engaging with the telepathic hypothesis may require analysts to confront the hyper-complexity of psychic matter, a

> complexity that challenges the reductionist paradigms that separate subjectivity from objectivity.

So, the telepathy hypothesis then leads us to reconsider the most fundamental levels of symbolization and the profound nature of the real. As Mayer (2001) notes:

> Our growing focus on what has been called the intersubjective nature of the analytic relationship will open up our investigations, leading us to a better understanding not only of conventional intersubjective reality, but also of the less conventional, certainly equally intersubjective, sphere of "telepathy" and other possibly anomalous perceptions.
>
> (p. 633)

By introducing the telepathic hypothesis into metapsychology, we are led to reconsider the boundaries of primary intersubjectivity, suggesting that certain interactions between analyst and analysand may reach beyond the conventional bounds of intersubjectivity, revealing something "beyond" the immediate, here-and-now experience (Tennes, 2007). Following the work of Djohar Si Amed (2006), who has theorized about telepathic process for many years, we can analyze telepathy in its relation to different levels of symbolization as illustrated in Figure 13.1 (Rabeyron, 2020a; Rabeyron et al., 2021):

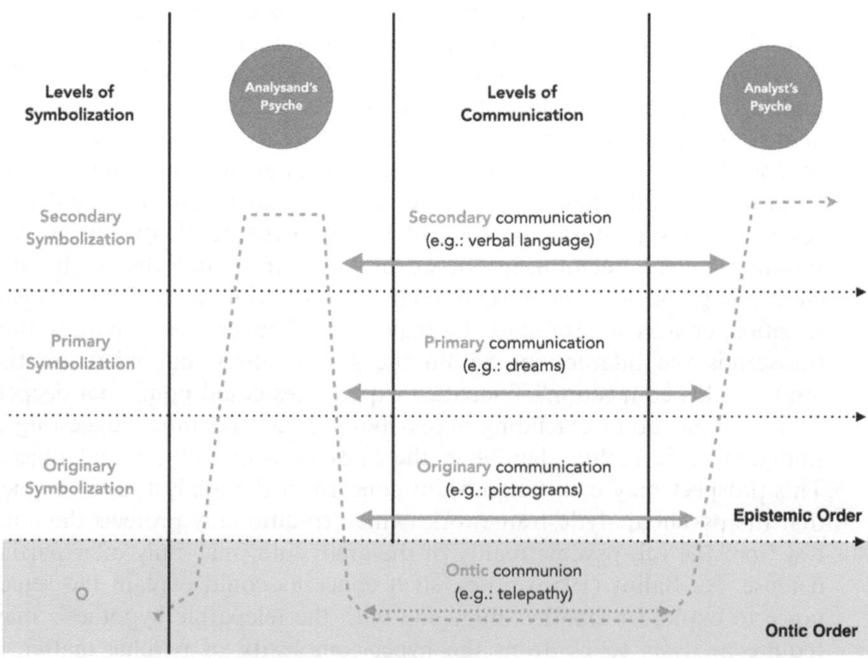

Figure 13.1 Telepathy and symbolization processes.

The left column outlines stages in the process of symbolization (original, primary, secondary) stemming from the O, emphasizing the progression of subjectivation that leads to the emergence of conscious thoughts. This process of subjectivation occurs progressively, with each stage marking a deeper structuring of the psyche. The line under the analysand's psyche illustrates how this process unfolds through various channels—verbal, nonverbal, pictorial, and ontic—within the dynamic of transference during analysis. Ontic communication is situated at the level of O, representing a form of interaction more fundamental than pictorial representations, and from which telepathic processes are hypothesized to emerge.

This process of the emergence of thought from the O partly explains why the content of telepathic experiences is usually expressed metaphorically, mirroring the mechanisms of dream work. This process of deformation can be understood as the consequence of the passage from the O to the different levels of symbolization. For example, it may lead to a disjunction between affect (of fear concerning a relative, for example) and representation (which has been the object of different forms of transformations), which necessitates interpretative work, as Freud proposed in several of his writings on telepathy. This transformative process of deformation highlights the primary nature of telepathic intuitions, which, when viewed through the lens of secondary processes, may become distorted or difficult to identify. Consequently, these intuitions may remain undetected within the analytical process, challenging the analyst's ability to grasp their full significance. Such a model also suggests the necessity for psychoanalysts to consider a primordial dimension of communication and integrate it more holistically into psychoanalytic metapsychology and clinical practice. By acknowledging this level of communication, analysts could expand their interpretive frameworks to account for the complex, often subtle, manifestations of telepathic phenomena and their role in the therapeutic relationship.

Dual-Aspect Decompositional Monism and the Orpheus Model

We need nevertheless to go further and propose a comprehensive model that could provide a more general framework for understanding telepathy. In this regard, the Orpheus model, which we will now describe in general terms, aims to understand the nature of "ontic level" above-mentioned and, more generally, psi phenomena like telepathy (Rabeyron, 2023).[2] This model has been inspired by the ideas of many philosophers, in particular Plato, Leibniz, Spinoza, Kant, Hegel, but also Whitehead, Schopenhauer, and Bergson. It also has its origins in several theories developed in the field of parapsychology, in particular the *Model of Pragmatic Information* (Lucadou, 1995) and the *General Quantum Theory* (Atmanspacher et al., 2002; Filk & Römer, 2011). But the main inspiration of this model is the Pauli–Jung conjecture (Pauli & Jung, 1952) and in particular its formalization by the philosopher and physicist Harald Atmanspacher (Atmanspacher, 2023; Atmanspacher & Fuchs, 2014; Atmanspacher & Rickles, 2022). Atmanspacher has used the mathematical formalism of quantum physics to model the principles identified by Jung and Pauli, based on the idea that "quantum entanglement gives us a lesson that we might be able to apply more globally to the mind–matter relationship" (Atmanspacher, 2018; p. 533).[3] This conjecture leads us to rethink the relationship between psyche and matter in a general manner, which is necessary to understand what telepathy really is. The Orpheus model is also in the footsteps of several psychoanalysts, in particular Freud, Jung, Lacan, Bion, and Eisenbud. In many respects, this model attempts to explore some of Bion's (1965) intuitions to their limits and therefore might be considered as a post-Bionian model (Rabeyron, 2019).

We are going to outline the global architecture of this model before explaining how telepathy could be more intelligible through it. This model corresponds philosophically to a "dual-aspect decompositional monism": "monism" because it assumes that mind and matter derive from the same substance; "decompositional" because it is decomposed from a single substance (unlike so-called "compositional" models); "dual-aspect" because this substance is approached from two aspects, two complementary perspectives (mind and matter). Such an approach had already inspired psychologists like Gustav Fechner, who explained as early as 1851: "Body and mind, or material and spiritual, or physical and psychic, are not different according to their foundation or essence, but only because of the difference in the point of view from which they are conceived or observed." More recently, philosophers Thomas Nagel and David Chalmers have expressed positions critical of physicalism and reductionism that are also in line with dual-aspect monism. In particular, Nagel (1974), in his famous article "What Is It Like to Be a Bat?" emphasized the profoundly irreducible nature of the subjective experience of a living being. As for David Chalmers (2007), he called the enigmatic nature of the phenomenal experience of consciousness the "hard problem" of consciousness. According to him, its source is an informational matrix from which consciousness and matter derive according to a "dual aspect principle."

As already evoked, dual-aspect monism has also been developed within the framework of the Pauli–Jung conjecture (1952) and better formalized by Atmanspacher (Atmanspacher, 2023; Atmanspacher & Rickles, 2022). In this conjecture, mind and matter represent two "epistemic" aspects of an underlying "ontic order" that is neither psychic nor physical. This order is considered to be "neutral" or "psycho-physical" and hence psychophysically neutral. Mind and matter, which constitute the "epistemic order," are considered as the two sides of the same coin, which is why there is a kind of parallelism between thought and brain activity. But this parallelism does not mean that thoughts emerge from neuronal activity (reductionism) nor that neuronal activity emerges from the thoughts (idealism).

This type of monism is called decompositional because the passage from the ontic order to the epistemic order operates like a prism that "breaks down" the ontic order into several elements in the epistemic order. Like in a kaleidoscope, an object (in this ontic order) is "decomposed" into several images (in the epistemic order).[4] When an object in front of a kaleidoscope is moved or modified, all the facets seen in it are instantly transformed. So, when one facet is transformed, so are the others. However, there is no direct causal relationship between the different facets. The same applies to the relationship between mind and matter: They correspond to two "facets" of the ontic order with no direct causal link. Concretely, if the neuronal activity changes, the thinking changes. And if the thinking changes, so does my neuronal activity. But this "co-relation" or "co-variance" is not a causal relationship.

I have proposed to represent such a model as a circle made up of three parts, delimited by a horizontal and a vertical axis (Figure 13.2) (Rabeyron, 2023). The two axes correspond to two "cuts." On the horizontal plane, the "epistemo-ontic cut" or "Kantian cut" derives from Kant's distinction between noumena and phenomena (Atmanspacher, 2023). The former correspond to "the thing-in-itself" and are immanent. This cut distinguishes between the world-in-itself (the real; the ontic order), which is accessible and representable only through our cognitive experience, and certain a priori categories of understanding (reality; the epistemic world). Vertically, the "psychophysical cut" or "Cartesian cut"

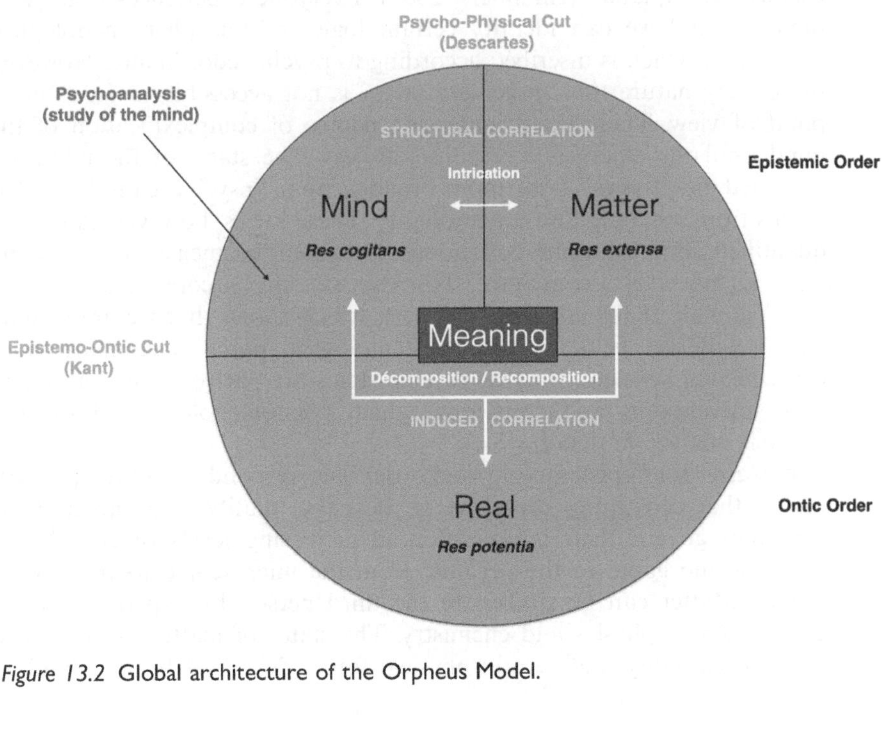

Figure 13.2 Global architecture of the Orpheus Model.

corresponds to René Descartes' distinction between mind (*Res Cogitans*) and matter (*Res Extensa*) (Atmanspacher, 2023). The former corresponds to psychic states experienced in the first person, while the latter refers to states of matter. These two "matters" derive from a more fundamental substance that makes up the ontic order, and which can be referred to as *Res Potentia*, as proposed by the physicist Werner Heisenberg.

The different parts delimited by these two cuts are organized by two types of relationships. First is the relationship vectorized by the process of decomposition–recomposition (or projection-feedback), which lies between the ontic order (the real) and the epistemic order (the reality). It corresponds to a decomposition of the ontic order in the form of the epistemic order. Transformations of the epistemic order in turn induce automatically transformations of the ontic order, according to a logic of "recomposition." The second process corresponds to the relationship between mind and matter according to a process of "entanglement" or "synchronicity" as called by Pauli and Jung (1952), a consequence of the decomposition process. Three main categories can thus be identified in this model—mind, matter, and the real—that we are now going to describe in more detail before explaining how to understand telepathy with this model.

1 The *Mind* (or "epistemic-psychic order") corresponds to all subjective experiences in the first person and takes the form of what philosophers usually call "qualia" (Chalmers, 2007). Everyone experiences it at every moment, and we can identify certain logics of this phenomenological experience, which is inscribed according to psychic coordinates. However, by its very nature this "psychic matter" is not accessible to an external point of view. There is an increasing degree of complexification of the mind until the emergence of consciousness. The states of the mind are governed by "forces" and, more broadly, by a "psychic causality" that comes from meaning and intentionality. These logics, however, cannot be quantified. For example, consciousness cannot be measured by saying "this person is 30% conscious." Nor can we "cut" a concept in half (for example, half of the concept of water), which shows that we are dealing with a different field from an epistemological point in comparison of experimental sciences. Finally, psychic states are part of emergent logics, both unconscious and conscious, which phenomenology and psychoanalysis analyze in detail.
2 The *Matter* (or "epistemo-physical order") corresponds to all the physical matter that constitutes the universe. It is the totality of atoms and the laws that govern their organization in increasing levels of complexity, from the inorganic to the organic, from the microscopic to the macroscopic. Matter can be studied in the third person by experimental sciences, such as physics and chemistry. The states of matter are governed by local causality and certain physical forces described by the standard

model forces (strong, weak, electromagnetic, gravitational). We can also identify certain limits or laws of matter, such as the speed of light and Planck's constant. The description of matter, at the macroscopic level, obeys the principle of non-contradiction and is expressed in the form of propositions, in particular Boolean algebra.[5]

3 The *Real* (or "ontic order") is not directly accessible by its very nature, and so its structure and lawful characteristics can only be induced indirectly through experience of coincident psyche and matter. "Psychic matter" and "physical matter" thus represent "emergences" from the real through the process of decomposition. Both immanent and transcendent, it is not governed by time, space, and causality as we know them. Nor is it organized by the principle of non-contradiction, and it corresponds to an infinite reservoir of possibilities. It cannot be represented, because our thinking necessarily follows finite spatio-temporal and causal coordinates. As Bion (1965) puts it, we can't think the real in the same manner that "we can't sing potatoes." While the ontic order cannot be cognitively apprehended, it can nevertheless be experienced through so-called "a-categoric" mystical experiences, which are considered to be "states that are experienced without conceptual or categorical content" (Atmanspacher, 2020, p. 12). In the psychoanalytic tradition, several authors have proposed terms to describe the real:[6] Sigmund Freud speaks of "the thing-in-itself," in reference to Kant; Jung proposed calling this world the *Unus Mundus* or the "Psychoid"; Lacan uses the term *real* in reference to Hegel's absolute.

Once we have described the global architecture of this model, we can distinguish two types of relationships between mind and matter, as proposed by Atmanspacher and Fach (2019):

1 *Structural correlations* correspond to the correlation of mind and matter according to an acausal logic based on the decomposition of the ontic order. These correlations link mental and cerebral states. They are stable, reproducible correlations, creating a *baseline of* the relationship between mind and matter, enabling them to be studied empirically in medicine and neurosciences.
2 *Induced correlations* take the form of direct "entanglements" between mind and matter as "signifying correspondences" or "psycho-physical correlations," what Jung and Pauli called "synchronicities."[7] These entanglements, which occur according to logics of meaning (Connolly, 2015), arise from the ontic order and do not correspond to a causal relationship in which the cause precedes the consequence. They take the form of "deviations" from structural correlations that occur occasionally, transiently, and are non-replicable. Atmanspacher (2020) notes that these "deviations are often represented as anomalies, paranormal, psychic or psi" (p. 10).

Telepathy would thus correspond to these induced correlations. They would be the consequence of interactions between mental states and matter states via the ontic order. We can think of them as "contraband" correlations that are supported by the ontic order and emancipated from the usual laws of time and space that organize the epistemic order. These induced correlations are deviations from structural correlations, and if there are no structural correlations, there can be no induced correlations. In other words, if there are no local (classical) correlations, there can be no non-local (psi) correlations. Psi (induced correlations) therefore tends to "deviate" or "twist" the stable relations of the epistemic order (structural correlations).

Any transformation in the epistemic order also has an automatic retroactive impact on the ontic order from which the epistemic order emerges. This reciprocal relationship induces a form of malleability in the real, which by its very nature makes it difficult to objectify. To put it another way, there is an inversely proportional relationship between the expression of psi (and telepathy) and its stability, which leads to the fact that these phenomena are elusive.

To illustrate this model, let us return to the case of Marion introduced at the beginning of this chapter. Marion experiences a sudden pain in her chest at the moment her mother dies of a heart attack. Following double-aspect decompositionnel models, mind and matter are linked by structural correlations that are stable and reproducible. This means that our thoughts and sensations are associated with measurable neural processes according to conventional physical laws. However, Marion's experience does not fit within such structural correlations: her body and emotional distress about her mother's passing, without any conventional channel of communication being involved. This experience is a temporary "deviation" from structural correlations and takes the form of a synchronicity, meaning a meaningful coincidence between Marion's psychological state and the tragic event experienced by her mother. This type of correlation does not rely on a traditional cause-and-effect relationship but rather on an "interconnection" at the level of the ontic order, a fundamental level disregarding conventional laws of time and space. In this particular case, due to their strong affective bond and the unconscious intentionality of Marion to save her mother, Marion experiences her mother's physical suffering, thereby taking the form of a connection beyond space and time. This experience illustrates how telepathy, within this model, is considered as a form of "non-local correlation" or "psychophysical entanglement" that arises from the ontic order.

Orpheus and the Principle of Elusiveness

As we have already mentioned, psi and telepathy are characterized by their elusive nature. Telepathic perceptions are almost systematically subject to distortions of the same kind as those found in dreams,[8] and the telepathic message usually appears encrypted or the phenomena are sporadic and occasional (as in the different clinical cases evoked at the beginning of this chapter). Consequently, there is no "telepathic radio" or "telepathic communication" as we can see in science-fictions movies, and we don't observe telepathic communications with the reliability of a phone communication or like a direct connection from mind to mind.[9]

While proponents of the "classical" or "Rhinean" experimental approach in parapsychology usually reject this elusive aspect of psi (Radin, 2010, 2018; Tressoldi & Storm, 2025), we believe it is essential to take into account elusiveness at a theoretical level, just as transference was initially considered an obstacle in psychoanalysis before being placed at the center of its theorization and practice. This elusiveness aspect is indeed so common that it is one of the most reproducible features of psi research, as already noted by Eisenbud (1966), who also remarks that the investigation of this elusive dimension had not been explored as much as it should have been. It is usually considered to be the consequence of the fact that psi has not yet been sufficiently understood to be replicable in a reliable manner. But Eisenbud considers elusiveness to be an intrinsic property of psi, as well as Arthur Koestler (1977), who explains:

> It's as if the phenomena in question leave a smokescreen in their wake to confuse those who try to identify them. This puzzling reaction is so widespread that it deserves a name. We could call it the cuttlefish effect, after the mollusk that casts a cloud of black ink when it knows it is under attack.
>
> (p. 9)

It is therefore necessary to integrate this elusive dimension to a global theory of psi as proposed in the Orpheus model. Referring to a myth is not insignificant, since myths express certain properties of the real in a condensed and metaphorical way. Like dreams, myths lie at the interface of the real and provide cryptic keys to understanding human nature. In this respect, the myth of Orpheus is particularly instructive for understanding psi and telepathy. Orpheus was a hero of Greek mythology, renowned for his gifts as a poet and musician. Known for his ability to charm animals and men with his lyre, he married Eurydice but, on their wedding day, she died after being bitten by a snake. Orpheus then tries to rescue her from the underworld, which Hades accepts with the condition that she remains silent and that Orpheus does not turn back until they have left the realm of the dead. Just as he is about to save his beloved, Orpheus is seized by a doubt and looks at Eurydice to be sure that she is behind him. Eurydice then disappears forever, and Orpheus is torn to pieces by the Bacchae, who do not want him to remain faithful to Eurydice even after his death.

We could interpret the myth in this way. The world of the dead and the world of the living would reflect the distinction between the real (ontic order) and reality (epistemic order), separated by a reputedly impassable barrier represented by the Acheron. Orpheus has a special relationship with the real, thanks to his talents as a poet and musician, and it is through his lyre that he manages to convince Hades. Orpheus is thus able to penetrate the real and attempt to "extract" Eurydice back to reality. But this requires tolerating a form of doubt and uncertainty that leads to accepting not seeing and not knowing. The myth would thus be a metaphor of the elusive aspect we have described before and more generally of what I have proposed to call the "principle of elusiveness" (Rabeyron, 2023). Psi cannot be used as a signal or directly observed at the risk of disappearing, just as Orpheus makes Eurydice disappear when he tries to verify her presence. This desire would be more archaic than Oedipal desire, and its transgression would lead to the worst punishments, symbolized here by the death of Eurydice. So, just as the Oedipus complex will be resolved by the integration of the prohibition of incest, the Orpheus complex will be resolved by the integration of a relationship to uncertainty or what Bion (1965) has called "negative capability." It represents a more primary form of limit in the relationship with the real: Human beings have to accept there are things they cannot see and cannot know.

In the case of telepathy, the principle of elusiveness takes more precisely the form of the "non-transmission axiom," as coined by Lucadou et al. (2007), according to which "entanglement relations cannot be used to transmit a signal or generate causal influences" (p. 17).[10] This is a consequence of the fact that any attempt to use a "non-local correlation" as a signal will result in the disappearing or a transformation of that non-local correlation in the system studied (Lucadou & Wald, 2014). From this point of view, a system is like an egg closed by a shell. It is possible to maintain a psi effect (or a telepathic connection) as long as the "organizational closure" is not broken by an external observer (i.e., as long as the egg is not cracked to see what is inside). When this is the case, psi entanglements diminish and gradually disappear, like the yolk flowing out of the egg once its shell has been broken. This explains why measuring or observing psi effects tends to make them disappear. It also explains why the analytical setting is perfect to produce telepathic phenomenon. The analyst–analysand dyad represents a closed "egg" whose intimacy prevents any form of objectification and thus catalyzes entanglement phenomena within the ontic order.[11]

Another consequence of the elusiveness principle is that it makes it tricky, if not impossible, to pinpoint the "source" of psi, and when this source is brought to light, it seems to dry up. For example, for a telepathic experience, we cannot know precisely where the information comes from (from the future? From the mind of the other person? As a clairvoyant perception?). We can therefore only make "close circles" around the source of psi without ever reaching it, as Jule Eisenbud (1966) already suggested. Bertrand Méheust (2015), for his part, assumes that the source of psi is like the crater of a volcano that can only be circled. This gives the impression that there is a "magic box" where psi comes from, a kind of umbilical cord to the real—an *omphalos*, as the Greeks called it—that we cannot grasp directly, at the risk of destroying such interactions. It therefore seems possible to observe and even partially objectify the effects of psi but not its source.

To Conclude: What Telepathy Is and What Telepathy Is Not

Telepathic phenomena belong to the broader category of psi perceptions[12] that correspond to specific interactions called "non-local." They indicate the existence of an "ontic order" within which the ordinary laws of space, time, and causality do not operate in the way we usually experience them. Such experiences occur spontaneously, but also within the analytical framework that potentiates such interactions. Thus, telepathy cannot be reduced to phenomena like projective identification or co-thinking processes. There is indeed an ontological valence and a "veridical" aspect in certain telepathic experiences. It is then possible to study these telepathic experiences from their various psychic functions in the analytical setting.

On a more theoretical level, certain difficulties arise when we try to understand the nature of such interactions. In this regard, it is important to understand that telepathy is not a transfer of information in the form of a signal like those studied in physics, which explains the difficulties encountered when trying to objectify telepathy in experimental conditions. Researchers then repeatedly encounter the elusive nature of these phenomena (Rabeyron, 2020b), which accounts for the fact that they primarily correspond to process associated with meaning and intentionality.[13] Telepathy should rather be understood as a form of "communion" in the ontic order, whose trace we then find in the epistemic order that organizes our subjective experience. It then offers a glimpse into the profound nature of the real and its interconnected dimension.

Notes

1 We will not address in this chapter Freud's historical writings on the theme of telepathy, nor his interest in psychic research. We refer the reader interested in this topic to Rabeyron et al. (2020). For an analysis of the correspondence between Freud and Ferenczi on this theme, we refer to Rabeyron and Evrard (2012) and Gyimesi (2012).

2 We can only describe this model in general terms in this chapter, and we apologize to the reader if certain points are only addressed partially and remain obscure. A more detailed description of this model is available in Rabeyron (2023).

3 If this formalism adopts the formalism of quantum physics, it does not lead to considering psi phenomena and telepathy as quantum phenomena.

4 This effect of decomposition can be seen during telepathy experiments with the "scattering phenomenon" described by psychiatrist Jan Ehrenwald (1978). The same phenomenon is illustrated, for example, by the classical experiments of Warcollier (1921) and, more recently, the work of Djohar Si Ahmed (1990, 2006, 2014), in which the "target" sent telepathy is "received" in a decomposed manner.

5 Boolean algebra, introduced by mathematician George Boole in 1854, distinguishes and operates on logical variables taking two states in particular: 0 (false) and 1 (true). We can then perform a number of operations and calculations on these variables and model different forms of logical reasoning in this way.

6 We may note that most cultures have developed a form of representation of the real that underpins the existence of reality. For example, the Sumerians evoke a "primordial sea," the Greeks call *Arché* the fundamental substance underlying reality, the Eleatics evoke the *Apeiron*, Parmenides speaks of the *Peiras*, and so on (Atmanspacher & Rickles, 2022). Eastern cultures, such as Hinduism, speak of *Brahman*, and we might also mention *the Dreamtime* of the Aborigines.

7 As Arthur Koestler (1972) notes, Jung borrowed the notion of synchronicity from Kammerer, a biologist working on acquired traits. In 1919, Kammerer published a work on the analysis of coincidences, and developed the idea of a "law of seriality" that would be "the umbilical cord linking thought, feeling, science and art to the bowels of the universe that gave birth to them" (p.?).

8 It should be noted in this regard that the distortions that characterize dreams could also be considered as the consequence of the transition from the ontic order (unconscious, infinite) to the epistemic order (conscious, finite).

9 However, there are cases where detailed information can still be obtained, such as the case of Alexis Didier (Méheust, 2003) or the Stargate Program (McMoneagle, 2002), but this always follows specific rules and conditions. For more details, see Rabeyron (2023).

10 There are, in fact, two types of elusiveness. The first, previously described, corresponds to transformation during the symbolization process. The second, a more fundamental form of elusiveness, arises from the transition from the ontic order to the epistemic order, a passage which is governed by the principle of elusiveness.

11 More generally, as Bion (1965) already observed, the analytic setting aims to bring forth "unthought thoughts" from O, and it is this fundamental process of embodying O that also generates telepathic phenomena between the analyst and analysand.

12 Indeed, it is not relevant to distinguish telepathy from clairvoyance or precognition, as these terms represent distinctions based on categories of space and time that organize the epistemic order, while, in reality, the source of these phenomena lies in the ontic order, which is not organized by such categories. Actually, there exists a unique psi process that manifests in different forms within its phenomenology in the epistemic order.

13 Telepathy cannot therefore be considered as a supposed quantum phenomenon, as this would place phenomena of a different nature within the physical realm. Considering telepathy as a quantum phenomenon is an epistemological error, as it leads to consider a phenomenon from the ontic order into the epistemic-physical order. However, quantum phenomena themselves also testify to this form of deep interconnection of reality, giving rise to "spooky action at a distance" between particles studied by physicists.

References

Alcock, J. E., Burns, J., & Freeman, A. (2003). *Psi wars: Getting to grips with the paranormal*. Imprint Academic.

Ansell, C. (1966). The unconscious: Agency of the occult. *Psychoanalytic Review*, 53, 164–171.

Anzieu, D. (1974). *Le moi-peau*. Dunod.

Anzieu, D. (1993). L'esprit, l'inconscient. *Nouvelle Revue de Psychanalyse*, 48, 149–162.
Atmanspacher, H. (2018). Synchronicity and the experience of psychophysical correlations. In C. Roesler (Ed.), *Research in analytical psychology* (pp. 227–242). Routledge.
Atmanspacher, H. (2020). The Pauli-Jung conjecture and its relatives: A formally augmented outline. *Open Philosophy*, 3, 527–549.
Atmanspacher, H. (2023). Why physics does not inform the human condition, but its boundaries do. *Foundations of Science*, 747, 1–13.
Atmanspacher, H., & Fach, W. (2019). Exceptional experiences of stable and unstable mental states, understood from a dual-aspect point of view. *Philosophies*, 4, 7–19.
Atmanspacher, H., & Fuchs, C. A. (2014). *The Pauli–Jung conjecture and its impact today.* Andrews UK.
Atmanspacher, H., & Rickles, D. (2022). *Dual-aspect monism and the deep structure of meaning*. Routledge.
Atmanspacher, H., Römer, H., & Walach, H. (2002). Weak quantum theory: Complementarity and entanglement in physics and beyond. *Foundations of Physics*, 32, 379–406.
Balint, M. (1955). Notes on parapsychology and parapsychological healing. *International Journal of Psychoanalysis*, 36, 31–35.
Bass, A. (2004). Imagine, I am a great soothsayer—the future is now: Commentary on Melanie Suchet's "Whose mind is it anyway?" *Studies in Gender and Sexuality*, 5, 303–316.
Bem, D. J., & Honorton, C. (1994). Does psi exist? Replicable evidence for an anomalous process of information transfer. *Psychological Bulletin*, 115, 4–18.
Bion, W. R. (1965). *Transformations: Change from learning to growth.* Heinemann.
Birot, É. (2016). Le transfert de pensée de l'homme aux loups à M. P. *Revue Française de Psychanalyse*, 81, 1626–1631.
Branfman, T. G., & Bunker, H. A. (1952). Three extrasensory perception dreams. *Psychoanalytic Quarterly*, 21, 190–195.
Brottman, M. (2011). *Phantoms of the clinic: From thought-transference to projective identification*. Karnac.
Cardeña, E. (2018). The experimental evidence for parapsychological phenomena: A review. *American Psychologist*, 73, 663–677.
Cardeña, E., Lynn, S. J., & Krippner, S. (2000). *Varieties of anomalous experience: Examining the scientific evidence.* American Psychological Association.
Cardeña, E., Palmer, J., & Marcusson-Clavertz, D. (2015). *Parapsychology: A handbook for the 21st century.* McFarland.
Chalmers, D. (2007). The hard problem of consciousness. In S. Schneider & M. Velmans (Eds.), *The Blackwell companion to consciousness* (pp. 32–41). Wiley-Blackwell.
Chaperot, C. (2011). Phénomènes d'allure télépathique dans la relation thérapeutique avec des patients schizophrènes: Hypothèse d'une potentielle nocivité de la pensée soignante. *Evolution Psychiatrique*, 76, 273–286.
Chervet, B. (2009). L'après-coup. *Revue Française de Psychanalyse*, 73, 1361–1441.
Connolly, A. (2015). Bridging the reductive and the synthetic: Some reflections on the clinical implications of synchronicity. *Journal of Analytical Psychology*, 60, 159–178.
Delanoy, D. (2005). Meta-analyses. In J. Henry (Ed.), *Parapsychology: Research on exceptional experiences* (pp. 42–62). Routledge.
De M'Uzan, M. (1977). *De l'art à la mort.* Gallimard.

de Peyer, J. (2014). Telepathic entanglements: Where are we today? Commentary on paper by Claudie Massicotte. *Psychoanalytic Dialogues*, 24, 109–121.

de Peyer, J. (2016). Uncanny communication and the porous mind. *Psychoanalytic Dialogues*, 26, 156–174.

de Peyer, J. (2017). Traversing the ineffable: Commentary on Sharon Farber's "Becoming a telepathic tuning fork." *Psychoanalytic Dialogues*, 27, 735–740.

Ehrenwald, J. (1971). Mother–child symbiosis: Cradle of ESP. *Psychoanalytic Review*, 58, 455–466.

Ehrenwald, J. (1978). *The ESP experience: A psychiatric validation*. Basic Books.

Eisenbud, J. (1966). *The world of Ted Serios: "Thoughtographic" studies of an extraordinary mind*. William Morrow.

Eisenbud, J. (1970). *Psi and psychoanalysis*. Grune & Stratton.

Eshel, O. (2006). Where are you, my beloved? On absence, loss, and the enigma of telepathic dreams. *International Journal of Psychoanalysis*, 87, 1603–1627.

Eshel, O. (2010). Patient–analyst interconnectedness: Personal notes on close encounters of a new dimension. *Psychoanalytic Inquiry*, 30, 146–154.

Eshel, O. (2012). A beam of "chimeric" darkness: Presence, interconnectedness, and transformation in the psychoanalytic treatment of a patient convicted of sex offenses. *Psychoanalytic Review*, 99, 149–178.

Eshel, O. (2019). Would clinical psychoanalysis shy away from delving further into the unknown? On the mystery of telepathic dreams. *International Journal of Psychoanalysis*, 100, 608–610.

Farber, S. K. (2017). Becoming a telepathic tuning fork: Anomalous experience and the relational mind. *Psychoanalytic Dialogues*, 27, 719–734.

Fechner, G. T. (1851). *Zend-Avesta oder uber die Dinge des Himmels und des Jenseits: Vom Standpunkte der Naturbetrachtung*. Leopold Voss.

Filk, T., & Römer, H. (2011). Generalized quantum theory: Overview and latest developments. *Axiomathes*, 21, 211–220.

Freud, S. (1921). Psychoanalysis and telepathy. In G. Devereux (Ed.), *Psychoanalysis and the occult* (pp. 56–68). International Universities Press.

Freud, S. (1922). Dreams and telepathy. In G. Devereux (Ed.), *Psychoanalysis and the occult* (pp. 69–86). International Universities Press.

Freud, S. (1925). The occult significance of dreams. In G. Devereux (Ed.), *Psychoanalysis and the occult* (pp. 87–90). International Universities Press.

Freud, S. (1933). Dreams and the occult. In G. Devereux (Ed.), *Psychoanalysis and the occult* (pp. 91–109). International Universities Press.

Green, A. (1983) *Narcissisme de vie, narcissisme de mort*, Paris, Les Editions de Minuit, 2007.

Gyimesi, J. (2012). Sándor Ferenczi and the problem of telepathy. *History of the Human Sciences*, 25, 131–148.

Hann-Kende, F. (1953). On the role of transference and countertransference in psychoanalysis. In G. Devereux (Ed.), *Psychoanalysis and the occult* (pp. 158–167). International Universities Press.

Hartmann, E. (1991). *Boundaries in the mind: A new psychology of personality*. Basic Books.

Helm, F. L. (2018). Free association continues. *Psychoanalytic Inquiry*, 38, 446–456.

Kammerer, P. (1919). *Boundaries in the mind: A new psychology of personality*. Basic Books.

Koestler, A. (1972). *The roots of coincidence.* Random House.
Koestler, A. (1977). *Janus: A summing up.* Hutchinson.
Kohut, H. (1972). Thoughts on narcissism and narcissistic rage. *The Psychoanalytic Study of the Child,* 27, 360–400.
Lazar, S. G. (2001). Knowing, influencing, and healing: Paranormal phenomena and implications for psychoanalysis and psychotherapy. *Psychoanalytic Inquiry,* 21, 113–131.
Lévy, G. (2007). Le transfert de pensées en séance. *Le coq héron,* 191, 59–63.
Löfgren, L. B. (1968). Recent publications on parapsychology. *Journal of the American Psychoanalytic Association,* 16, 146–178.
Lucadou, W. (1995). The model of pragmatic information (MPI). *European Journal of Parapsychology,* 11, 58–75.
Lucadou, W., Römer, H., & Walach, H. (2007). Synchronistic phenomena as entanglement correlations in generalized quantum theory. *Journal of Consciousness Studies,* 14, 50–74.
Lucadou, W., & Wald, F. (2014). Extraordinary experiences in its cultural and theoretical context. *International Review of Psychiatry,* 26, 324–334.
Mayer, E. L. (2001). On "telepathic dreams?" An unpublished paper by Robert J. Stoller. *Journal of the American Psychoanalytic Association,* 49, 629–657.
Mayer, E. L. (2007). *Extraordinary knowing: Science, skepticism, and the inexplicable powers of the human mind.* Bantam.
McMoneagle, J. (2002). *The Stargate chronicles.* Hampton Roads Publishing.
Méheust, B. (1999). *Somnambulisme et mediumnité.* Les Empêcheurs de penser en rond.
Méheust, B. (2003). *Un voyant prodigieux: Alexis Didier, 1826–1866.* Les Empêcheurs de penser en rond.
Méheust, B. (2015). *Jesus thaumaturge.* InterEditions.
Nagel, T. (1974). What is it like to be a bat? *The Philosophical Review,* 83(4), 435–450.
Papazian, B. (2017). "Telepathic" phenomena and separation anxiety. *International Journal of Psychoanalysis,* 98, 1169–1192.
Pauli, W., & Jung, C. G. (1952). *The interpretation of nature and the psyche.* Princeton University Press.
Plas, R. (2000). *Naissance d'une science humaine, la psychologie: Les psychologues et le merveilleux psychique.* PUR.
Prados, M. (1959). Transference and seemingly parapsychological phenomena. *Psychoanalytic Review,* 46, 29–44.
Rabeyron, T. (2019). Transformational processes and the analytic field: A new paradigm for clinical models and practices. *L'Évolution Psychiatrique,* 85, 104–114.
Rabeyron, T. (2020a). *Clinique des expériences exceptionnelles.* Dunod.
Rabeyron, T. (2020b). Why most research findings about psi are false: The replicability crisis, the psi paradox and the myth of Sisyphus. *Frontiers in Psychology,* 11. doi:10.3389/fpsyg.2020.562992
Rabeyron, T. (2023). *Codex anomalia.* InterEditions.
Rabeyron, T., & Evrard, R. (2012). Perspectives historiques et contemporaines sur l'occulte dans la correspondance Freud-Ferenczi. *Recherches en Psychanalyse,* 13, 97–97.
Rabeyron, T., Evrard, R., & Massicotte, C. (2020). Psychoanalysis and the sour apple: Thought-transference in historical and contemporary psychoanalysis. *Contemporary Psychoanalysis,* 56, 612–652.

Rabeyron, T., Evrard, R., & Massicotte, C. (2021). Psychoanalysts and telepathic processes. *Journal of the American Psychoanalytic Association*, 69, 535–571.

Rabeyron, T., & Loose, T. (2015). Anomalous experiences, trauma, and symbolization processes at the frontiers between psychoanalysis and cognitive neurosciences. *Frontiers in Psychology*, 6. doi:10.3389/fpsyg.2015.01926

Rabeyron, T., & Watt, C. (2010). Paranormal experiences, mental health and mental boundaries, and psi. *Personality and Individual Differences*, 48, 487–492.

Radin, D. (2010). *The conscious universe: The scientific truth of psychic phenomena*. HarperEdge.

Radin, D. (2018). *Real magic*. Harmony.

Reichbart, R. (2019). *The paranormal surrounds us: Psychic phenomena in literature, culture and psychoanalysis*. McFarland.

Reiner, A. (2004). Psychic phenomena and early emotional states. *Journal of Analytical Psychology*, 49, 313–336.

Rhine-Feather, S., & Schmicker, M. (2005). *The gift: The extraordinary experiences of ordinary people*. St. Martin's.

Rizzolo, G. S. (2016). The critique of regression: The person, the field, the lifespan. *Journal of the American Psychoanalytic Association*, 64, 1097–1131.

Rosenbaum, R. (2011). Exploring the other dark continent: Parallels between psi phenomena and the psychotherapeutic process. *Psychoanalytic Review*, 98, 57–90.

Sánchez-Medina, A. (2018). Projective identification and "telepathic dreams". *International Journal of Psychoanalysis*, 99, 380–390.

Searles, H. F. (1979). *Countertransference and related subjects: Selected papers*. International Universities Press.

Servadio, E. (1935). Psychoanalyse und telepathie. *Imago*, 21, 489–497.

Servadio, E. (1958). Magic and castration-complex. *International Journal of Psychoanalysis*, 39, 147–150.

Si Ahmed, D. (1990). *Parapsychologie et psychanalyse*. Dunod.

Si Ahmed, D. (2006). *Comment penser le paranormal: Psychanalyse des champs limites de la psyché*. L'Harmattan.

Si Ahmed, D. (2014). *Pour une psychanalyse des expériences exceptionnelles*. L'Harmattan.

Storm, L., Tressoldi, P., & Risio, L. D. (2010). Meta-analysis of free-response studies, 1992–2008: Assessing the noise reduction model in parapsychology. *Psychological Bulletin*, 136, 471–485.

Tennes, M. (2007). Beyond intersubjectivity. *Contemporary Psychoanalysis*, 43, 505–525.

Thalbourne, M. A. (2000). Transliminality: A review. *International Journal of Parapsychology*, 11, 1–34.

Tressoldi, P., & Storm, L. (2025). The myth of the decline effect in psi research: The empirical evidence. *Journal of Scientific Exploration*, in press.

Ullman, M., Krippner, S., & Vaughan, A. (1973). *Dream telepathy*. Hampton Roads Publishing.

Warcollier, R. (1921). *La télépathie-recherches expérimentales*. Félix Alcan.

Widlöcher, D. (1996). *Les nouvelles cartes de la psychanalyse*. Odile Jacob.

Wiseman, R. (2010). Heads I win, tails you lose: How parapsychologists nullify null results. *Skeptical Inquirer*, 34, 36–39.

Conclusion

Richard Reichbart

We have tried in this collection to provide in-depth clinical articles about telepathy, replete with specific details of how a patient's dreams or communications coincided strikingly with a dream or event in the analyst's life, and we have explicated the dynamic aspects of these telepathic communications. In addition, in many of these chapters we have traced the history of telepathy in psychoanalytic thought, beginning with Freud and Ferenczi. And then across various psychoanalytic orientations—Freudian, Winnicotian, Bionian, Relational—we have expressed the hope that psychoanalysts will embrace the importance of telepathy in its transference and countertransference manifestations, as a way of deepening the patient's treatment. Last, many of us have opened the window further by speaking of psychic phenomena beyond telepathy and by exploring the scientific implications of the telepathic phenomenon.

We can only hope that this book is a fitting continuation of such work as Devereux's 1953 collection *Psychoanalysis and the Occult*. Whether one believes the compelling perspective of Ofra Eshel, who presents cases of patients who have had losses in their development, that led to their need to telepathically keep in touch with and reach their psychoanalyst in the present, or the beliefs of Thomas Rayberon, Karen Peoples, Richard Reichbart, Janine de Peyer, Mikita Brottman, Ruth Rosenbaum and others that telepathy occurs beyond just these patients, all of us, regardless of our belief, unanimously and staunchly contend that psychoanalysts should follow in the footsteps of Freud, who believed that telepathy existed. Rather than avoiding or minimizing or discounting the telepathic hypothesis, as has been all too common in establishment psychoanalysis, psychoanalysts should be glad to explore the hypothesis. One can see by reading these chapters, telepathy in the clinical process can reveal much, in poignant terms, about the "true" relationship between analyst and patient.

As we have indicated, as striking as they are, there is actually nothing *factually* new in these wonderful accounts. Such accounts—as in Devereux's compilation—have existed since the beginning of psychoanalysis. What *is* new here are the theoretical formulations as to why telepathy exists in psychoanalysis (and in our lives), formulations so notable that we hope they gain traction in the

DOI: 10.4324/9781003611042-15

psychoanalytic and parapsychological scientific universes. For that matter, although historically this has always been problematic, it would be felicitous if this book helped bring those two universes closer together.

Freud began his adventure by wondering repeatedly about the nature of psychological process—about how dreams formed, about the nature and effect of development, about the twists and turns of transference and countertransference—and a century ago, he explored telepathy. We offer this book in furtherance of Freud's exploratory ethos, that powerful invocation by him of the need to question that is so central to the psychoanalytic endeavor with patients.

Reference

Devereux, G. (1953). *Psychoanalysis and the occult*. International Universities Press.

Index

For Product Safety Concerns and Information please contact our EU representative GPSR@taylorandfrancis.com Taylor & Francis Verlag GmbH, Kaufingerstraße 24, 80331 München, Germany